PERFECT 1

Copyright © .

DISCLAIMER

Contents

Preface

The creation of beauty is art.
- Ralph Waldo Emerson, American poet

Beauty is a creation. German philosopher Georg Wilhelm Friedrich Hegel said, "I'm not ugly, but my beauty is a total creation." So just like an artist requires the very best tools and skill to create a magnificent piece of artwork, a woman needs the very best beauty products and also skill to be a masterpiece of beauty.

I decided to write a product picks guide due to the fact that finding the very best products is not always easy. Advertisers claim to offer the best and yet many times fail to deliver results. Author Adam Osborne wisely said, "I'm a strict believer in the scientific principle of believing nothing."

My book, *How to Be a Perfect 10: Women's Guidebook to Increasing Attractiveness*, was intended to be a standard edition that excludes brand names since newer and better products are constantly being released. A product pick guide can be updated with the newest and best products every so often. However, if you want to keep as up-to-date as possible with the latest beauty products, subscribe to *Organic Spa Magazine* (www.organicspamagazine.com) and the magazine *New Beauty* (www.newbeauty.com).

Some of the information from my book, *How to Be a Perfect 10: Women's Guidebook to Increasing Attractiveness*, is included in this book as a refresher of the most important points and instructions on product usage and purchasing information.

The best way to find and purchase the picks in this book is to go to www.google.com and type the exact name of the product as it appears in this book. The Google search should bring up results of various online stores that sell the specific product.

My standards are simple: Only the best of the best. Life is too short to settle for anything less than the best! Off course to settle for the best, you must know what the best is. This book contains all the absolute best products currently available at press. Each product was selected based on thorough research and analysis.

The ingredients of each individual beauty product in this book have been analyzed to ensure its health safety because as the natural health community says, "If you can't eat it don't put it on your skin." Many of the product picks in this book have been evaluated for health safety at Environmental Working Group (www.ewg.org/skindeep). Environmental Working Group (EWG) rates products and ingredients, with a score of 0-2 (low hazard), 3-6 (moderate hazard), or 7-10 (high hazard). Approximately 99% of beauty product picks in this book have a EWG health score of 0-2 (low hazard). Many of the products have also received rave reviews and has been proven to be effective by many customers on review websites such as *Make Up Alley* (www.makeupalley.com).

Some women may be surprised to discover that the best products are not always the most expensive. Some companies simply price an item higher because of brand recognition even if the product is of poor quality or toxic in some way.

As with my first book, I must also mention the improvement of inner beauty. As American actress Priscilla Presley said, "Inner beauty should be the most important part of improving one's self." I have selected the very best products for improving inner beauty based on rave reviews.

Aiming at perfect 10 beauty is a goal of many women. There is nothing wrong with the pursuit of perfection in beauty. Just be careful to maintain a healthy level of perfectionism and avoid yourself from gravitating towards an unhealthy level of perfectionism. Healthy perfectionists are motivated, while unhealthy perfectionists are obsessed. Lord Chesterfield said, "Aim at perfection in everything, though in most things it is unattainable. However, they who aim at it, and persevere, will come much nearer to it than those whose laziness and despondency make them give it up as unattainable."

Healthy perfectionists understand that certain forms of imperfection are desirable because they are unique. Uniqueness is attractive, interesting, stimulating, and awe-inspiring. There is even something to be said about finding perfection in imperfection. As American author and poet Alice Walker once said, "In nature, nothing is perfect and everything is perfect. Trees can be contorted, bent in weird ways, and they're still beautiful."

Beauty icon Marilyn Monroe said, "Imperfection is beauty." Some female beauties have perfect imperfections: Eva Mendes little overbite, Kate Bosworth's two different colored eyes, Christina Ricci's large forehead and wide-set eyes, Gisele Bundchen's nose, Kate Moss' wide-set eyes, and Cindy Crawford's mole.

Chapter 1: Cosmetic Procedures

If somebody wants to have plastic surgery, more power to them.
- Shannen Doherty, American actress

The highest rated cosmetic facial procedures are Ultherapy and Invisalign. Invisalign straightens crooked teeth with a series of clear aligners that can be removed and are nearly invisible. Incognito Lite Braces is another newer option. Ultherapy uses ultrasound, which lifts, tones, and tightens loose skin on the face.

The highest rated cosmetic body procedure is Vaser Liposuction, which works to remove fat on the body. Cellulaze is rated an effective method of reducing cellulite.

This chapter does not list every single type of cosmetic procedure available, but rather, the most common and highest rated procedures.

The best place to find cosmetic surgeons is on www.ratemds.com and www.makemeheal.com/directory. To find out about cosmetic procedures go to www.realself.com and www.plasticsurgery.org.

TOP FACIAL PROCEDURES
Ultherapy
www.ultherapy.com

Invisalign
www.invisalign.com

TOP BODY PROCEDURES
Vaser Liposuction
www.vaser.com

Cellulaze
www.cellulaze.com

FACE

Rhinoplasty, also known as a "nose job," is one of the most common cosmetic procedures used to permanently minimize the size of the nose. Rhinoplasty has a high success rate. The most important factor that influences success is the right choice of rhinoplasty surgeon. Non-surgical rhinoplasty involves injecting skin fillers on different parts of the nose to fill in grooves and hide imperfections. This non-surgical procedure is not permanent.

Otoplasty, also called ear surgery, reshapes and repositions the ears to correct protruding and large ears. Incisions are made behind the ears and excess skin and soft tissue is trimmed away and the ears set closer to the head.

Dermal fillers such as Perlane, Restylane, Juvederm, and Prevelle are one of the simplest ways to increase beauty score ratings by simply increasing volume in certain areas of the face. These fillers can be used to plump up the cheeks, plump up lips, and fill facial lines.

Botox (botulinum toxin type A) works to relax the contraction of muscles by blocking nerve impulses. The result is muscles that can no longer contract, and so the wrinkles relax and soften. The effects tend to last from four to six months. Most patients require periodic reinjections to smooth out wrinkles and lines as they begin to reappear, but after each injection the wrinkles return less severely as the muscles are trained to relax. Botulinum toxin is very effective for women with frown lines, forehead creases, crow's feet, and platysmal bands on the neck.

Fraxel removes the top layers of skin to reveal a new layer of skin and stimulates collagen production. It is often used to treat wrinkles, sun damage, age spots, acne scarring, and skin discoloration. There are different types of Fraxel resurfacing treatments and each treatment has a slightly different recovery time and feels a little different.

The CO2 laser is a carbon dioxide laser used to resurface skin and treat discoloration, scars, warts, and enlarged pores, freckles, age spots, fines lines, and wrinkles.

A photofacial, also known as photorejuvination, is an intense pulsed light therapy to treat broken vapillaries, sun damage, enlarged pores, freckles, age spots, redness, rosacea, fine lines, and wrinkles.

V-Beam treats spider veins, warts, rosacea, psoriasis, scars, stretch marks, and birthmarks. It is a laser treatment that uses a cooling spray to help decrease the discomfort associated with treatment.

Photodynamic Therapy (PDT) treats sun damage, redness, flushing, discoloration, scars, and wrinkles. PDT uses a combination of a drug applied to the skin and a low intensity light system that activates the medication, killing sun damaged cells.

A face-lift involves fairly extensive surgery and works best for older women with loose, wrinkled, saggy skin. A woman can look at least ten years younger with a face-lift.

Venus Freeze tightens the skin and reduces wrinkles. The multi-polar radio frequency causes a thermal reaction in the tissue which stimulates the body's natural healing response. That restoring response causes new collagen to form, and the production of new elastin fibres.

A phenol peel is a deep chemical skin peel and is the strongest of all chemical peels. It treats wrinkles and major sun damage by peeling away the skin's top layers.

LaViv is product made from your own fibroblasts. It boosts collagen production. It is effective for fine lines especially around the eyes and lips.

Lower blepharoplasty reduces puffy bags under the eyes. Upper eyelid blepharoplasty is used to remove fat deposits, very loose skin, and drooping on the upper eyelids. Ultherapy will tighten and lift mild to moderate dropping of the upper eyelids.

Hairline lowering involves removing a section of the skin on the forehead and pulling the scalp forward, effectively shortening a high forehead.

Mentoplasty (chin reduction) will reduce the size of the chin to shorten a very long face. Shaving (burring) the chin bone will change the shape and size and a sliding genioplasty will reposition and reshape the chin point.

Submental liposuction removes fat from under the chin. It removes stubborn fat deposits, which do not respond to diet and exercise.

Ultherapy will tighten and lift mild to moderate loose or sagging skin on the jawline with ultra focused ultrasound energy waves.

Exilis is a non-invasive form of treatment for mild to moderate fat deposits. It is also effective for tightening the skin and reducing wrinkles.

A lower face-lift removes very loose, droopy skin on the jawline and tightens the bottom third of the face.

Mandible reduction will reduce the width of the jawline to make the lower face look narrower and thus more feminine. Mandible angle reduction will reduce the squareness near the back of the jawbone. In many cases, both these procedures are done together.

A neck lift will tighten sagging and loose neck skin, which is often called "Turkey neck". Neck liposuction is for women that have good neck elasticity and only excess fat to remove under the jawline on the neck. In some cases, a neck lift will need to be combined with neck liposuction.

The best way to get teeth cleaned and whitened at the dentist's office is with ultrasonic dental cleaning. It can prevent gingivitis, periodontal disease, and remove heavy stains.

Perhaps one of the most natural ways to whiten teeth is by use of dental ozone. Ozone sends activated oxygen below the enamel surface, much the same way as the teeth whitening bleaches. It has also been considered an effective way of treating cavities and other oral issues.

If ozone and ultrasound dental cleaning don't work to whiten teeth to a desirable shade then using a commercial teeth-whitening system is another option. However, many of these teeth-whitening systems are not the healthiest and best option. A study published in the *Journal of Dentistry* found that teeth lost some enamel hardness after the application of several different teeth-whitening products. Teeth-whitening systems, when used in excess, can weaken enamel. Weakened enamel can lead to tooth sensitivity, pain, gum irritation, and, in some cases, tooth decay. Dr. Shereen Azer, DDS, BDS, MS, MSC, says "People just have to understand that tooth whitening is not without side effects."

There are two main types of tooth discoloration: extrinsic and intrinsic discoloration. Extrinsic discoloration occurs in the outer layer of the tooth, called the enamel. Coffee, tea, colas, and wines can cause extrinsic tooth stains. Excessive fluoride also can cause teeth discoloration. Extrinsic staining can be effectively treated using a dentist-prescribed overnight bleaching. A study entitled, "Review of the effectiveness of various teeth whitening systems" published in *Operative Dentistry*, found that dentist-prescribed overnight bleaching with 10% carbamide peroxide (3.5% hydrogen peroxide) was shown to be the most effective method of teeth whitening. The second most effective system is placing the tooth whitening gel in a tray and using it during the daytime for shorter periods of time. In-office tooth whitening systems with 25%-40% hydrogen peroxide cause the teeth to become light immediately after bleaching. However, two weeks after completing in-office tooth whitening, it was found to be as effective as over-the-counter tooth whitening.

Scandinavian Institute of Dental Materials recommends avoiding the use of concentrations higher than 10% carbamide peroxide. A study entitled, "Effects of 10% carbamide peroxide on the enamel surface morphology" published in the *Journal of Esthetic and Restorative Dentistry* found that that 10% carbamide peroxide is fairly safe. The study showed that teeth whitening products with 10% carbamide peroxide cause erosion to the enamel immediately after bleaching, and the degree of erosion depends on the duration of application time. However, damage to the enamel reverts to almost normal within 3 months.

There are alternatives to non-peroxide based teeth whiteners. *Botanical White* is a teeth-whitening product that contains natural ingredients. It uses sodium bicarbonate micro crystals, which is an effective whitener that produces little or no teeth sensitivity.

There are simple ways to protect enamel during tooth whitening. Use remineralizing toothpaste. Use products with amorphous calcium phosphate such as *Arm & Hammer's* Enamel Care toothpaste. Chew xylitol gum containing funoran and calcium hydrogenphosphate. You can also use xylitol toothpaste gel such as *Now Foods* Xyli White Toothpaste Gel.

Intrinsic discoloration occurs in the inner structure of the tooth, called the dentin, when the dentin darkens or displays a yellow or gray tint. Intrinsic staining is more stubborn, and may require covering the tooth's outer surface with a color-matched composite bonding material, porcelain veneers or porcelain crowns. Composite resin veneers, which cost about $250 per tooth, are applied directly to your teeth and sculpted in the desired shape and shade. Porcelain veneers, which are thin porcelain shells bonded over the front of your teeth, cost over $900 per tooth. Porcelain crowns, also called caps, average $600 to $3,000 per tooth. Lumineers, made from Cerinate porcelain, costs over $700 per tooth.

Emmi-dent (www.emmi-dent.com) is the absolute best way currently available to clean the mouth and whiten the teeth. It is no-brushing toothbrush technology that uses 100% ultrasound to clean the teeth and gums by simply holding the brush next to the teeth for 8-10 seconds.

Emmi-dent generates ultrasound with a patented ultrasonic microchip that is embedded inside the brush head. This chip creates up to 96 million ultrasonic (air oscillations) impulses per minute and transmits them via the bristles and special nano-bubble toothpaste onto the teeth. *Emmi-dent* whitens the teeth, removes plaque and tarter, and kills bacteria in the mouth, under the gum, and in between the teeth. People have seen amazing stain-removing results and an improvement in the whiteness of the teeth. It may not produce excessively white Hollywood teeth, but it also doesn't damage the teeth.

MINIMIZE NOSE
Rhinoplasty
Non-Surgical Rhinoplasty

MINIMIZE EARS
Otoplasty

PLUMP CHEEKS / LIPS
Perlane
Juvederm
Restylane
Prevelle

REPAIR SKIN
Botox
Fraxel
CO2 Laser
Photofacial
V-Beam
Photodynamic Therapy
Facelift
Venus Freeze
Phenol Peel
Laviv

REDUCE FOREHEAD
Hair Line Lowering

TIGHTEN BROWS
Browlift

TIGHTEN EYELIDS
Blepharoplasty
Ultherapy

REDUCE CHIN
Mentoplasty
Submental Liposuction

TIGHTEN JAWLINE
Ultherapy

Exilis
Lower Face Lift

REDUCE JAWLINE
Mandible Reduction
Mandible Angle Reduction

TIGHTEN NECK
Neck Lift
Neck Liposuction

TEETH-WHITENING SERVICES
Ozone Teeth Whitening
Ultrasonic Teeth Cleaning

TEETH-WHITENING PRODUCTS
Opalescence Non-PF 10%
Colgate Platinum Professional System
Nite White ACP 10% Carbamide Peroxide
Botanical White
Arm & Hammer Whitening Booster
Eco-Dent ExtraBrite Tooth Whitener

BODY

A body lift is actually a combination of surgical procedures, usually a butt lift, bilateral thigh lifts and a tummy tuck. Body lifts are often done to remove and tighten up excess skin after a dramatic weight loss.
   Gastric bypass is a surgical procedure that permanently reroutes the digestive tract. It treats obesity by shrinking stomach capacity and a person's ability to overeat.
   Sleeve gastrectomy surgically reduces the size of the stomach permanently to about 25% of its original size. Sleeve gastrectomy limits the amount of food an individual can consume and helps them feel full sooner.
   A lap band is an inflatable band placed around the top portion of the stomach, shrinking its size. An individual then consume less food, resulting in weight loss.
   Women that are overweight can undergo tumescent liposuction. Tumescent liposuction, also referred to as liposculpture, uses small suction mechanism to target specific fat deposits under the skin. The procedure is used to contour or fine tune areas of the body. This procedure uses local anesthesia and has minimal downtime.
   Lipotherme is a minimally invasive procedure that uses a laser to liquefy and remove unwanted fat in targeted body zones. Lipotherme also tightens and firms the skin.
   SmartLipo and SlimLipo use a laser to heat up and liquefy unwanted fat, which is then removed from the body. SlimLipo laser therapy claims to melt away fat better than SmartLipo.

Liposonix uses high-intensity ultrasound energy and works well for reducing fat in the arms, thighs, and abdominal area. Liposonix may also work to tighten the skin.

CoolSculpting uses precisely controlled cooling to destroy fat cells. The typical amount of fat lost through CoolSculpting in a given area is about 20-25% percent per area treated.

Body Jet liposuction, also called Water Jet Liposuction, uses water pressure to remove body fat, without the pain and bruises found in standard liposuction procedures.

Abdominoplasty, also know as a "tummy tuck" surgically removes fat and excess, loose, hanging skin from the abdomen while also tightening the muscles resulting in a tighter looking abdomen. Panniculectomy is a similar procedure to abdominoplasty, except that it does not involve any muscle tightening.

Many who have lost weight through diet, exercise, or weight loss surgery (gastric bypass surgery) will be left with sagging skin on the arms. Brachioplasty, also known as an arm lift, is a surgical cosmetic procedure that reduces excess, sagging, loose skin and fat of the under portion of the upper arm.

Exilis is a non-invasive radio frequency treatment for reducing mild to moderate fat deposits and sagging skin on the arms.

As women age or have children, their breasts tend sag. Mastopexy, also known as a breast lift, removes excess skin to perk up sagging breasts.

Many who have lost weight through diet, exercise, and weight loss surgery will be left with sagging skin on the thighs. A thigh lift is a surgical procedure that reduces excess skin, and in some cases fat, on the inner or outer thighs.

A Brazilian Butt Lift is a type of buttock augmentation procedure, which removes fat from one area of the body and injects it into the buttocks to add volume and projection.

Labiaplasty is a cosmetic surgery procedure for altering the labia minora and the labia majora. It improves the size and appearance of the labia, which can become darkened, enlarged, and sagging from pregnancy or a number of other reasons.

Electrolysis is a hair removal method that uses an electrical current to destroy the hair root, dermal papilla, and hair germinating cells, ending further hair growth. It is a permanent option for the removal of hair, and works well to remove very fine and light-colored hair.

Intense Pulsed Light (IPL) and laser hair removal keep unwanted hairs away for a long time. The two methods are very similar. Laser hair removal uses a laser while IPL uses a light based device. Both procedures generate heat to damage and burn the hair follicles by the root. You can also purchase an at-home device for hair removal. The *Tria* laser is a laser home device, and *Silk'n SensEpil* is an IPL home device.

Sclerotherapy is a procedure used to treat unwanted blood vessels. A solution, called the sclerosing solution, is injected through a very fine needle, directly in to the veins. The sclerosing solution irritates the lining of the vessels, causing them to turn to scar tissue and eventually fade or disappear.

Asclera is an FDA-approved drug that treats spider veins by causing them to seal shut. The drug is injected at the site and is said to be painless.

Audrey Christian Venetrim is a cream that treats varicose and spider veins. The cream helps to strengthen blood vessels, reduce bruising and enhance blood circulation.

miraDry is a non-invasive treatment that reduces excessive sweating permanently. It uses microwave energy to shrink or entirely eliminate underarm sweat glands.

TIGHTEN FULL-BODY
Body Lift

MINIMIZE FAT
Gastric bypass
Sleeve Gastrectomy
Lap Band

REMOVE FAT
Tumescent Liposuction
Lipotherme
SmartLipo / SlimLipo
Liposonix
CoolSculpting
Body Jet

TIGHTEN ABDOMINALS
Abdominoplasty
Panniculectomy

TIGHTEN ARMS
Brachioplasty
Exilis

TIGHTEN BREASTS
Mastopexy

TIGHTEN THIGHS
Thigh Lift

PLUMP BUTTOCKS
Brazilian Butt Lift

REDUCE LABIA
Labiaplasty

REMOVE BODY HAIR
Electrolysis
Laser Hair Removal
Intense Pulsed Light

REMOVE BLOOD VESSELS
Sclerotherapy
Asclera
Audrey Christian Venetrim

REMOVE BODY ODOR
miraDry

Chapter 2: Makeup

That's the mistake women make - you shouldn't see your makeup.
We don't want to look like we've made an effort.
- Lauren Hutton, American model

All selected makeup products in this chapter are natural and even
beneficial to the skin, lips, and nails. The best place to find and purchase
the selected makeup products in this chapter is on www.amazon.com or
specific brand websites.

TOP MAKEUP BRANDS
Zosimos Botanicals
www.zosimosbotanicals.com

Gourmet Body Treats
www.gourmetbodytreats.com

Delizioso Skincare
www.deliziososkincare.com

100% Pure
www.100percentpure.com

Lauren Brooke Cosmetiques
www.laurenbrookecosmetiques.com

Au Naturale Cosmetics
www.aunaturaleglow.com

Vapour Organic Beauty
www.vapourbeauty.com

SKIN MAKEUP

Some women are not sure whether to use foundation or concealer first. Make up artist and beauty expert Cynde Watson says, "If your face feels naked without foundation, apply it first. Then dot concealer only where you need extra coverage."

Begin by applying a primer all over your face. Liquid foundation is best applied in a patting motion using a stippling brush to achieve flawless looking, airbrushed skin. Liquid foundation can also be applied with fingers. All the great makeup artists agree that clean fingers are a good way to apply liquid foundation. Apply liquid foundation on your face all the way into your hairline and on your neck so there is no "mask" of foundation. Then apply a concealer on areas with visible skin imperfections. You can then apply a bronzer on your face to give a tanned appearance or to contour your face. To add a glow to your face, apply an illuminator on the tops of your cheekbones and brow bone. Complete your look with finishing powder lightly dusted on your face. Then to set your powder, apply a light mist of thermal water facial spray.

Retractable makeup brushes are the most convenient because they don't make a powdery mess, and for avid travelers or women on the go they can be thrown into your purse.

PRIMER
Gourmet Body Treats Foundation Primer
Delizioso Skincare Pure Primer
Maia's Mineral Galaxy Liquid Primer
Zosimos Botanicals Unscented Primer
100% Pure Luminous Primer
Garden Botanika Skin Rejuvenating Face Treatment
JaDora Cosmetics Skin Primer
Vapour Organic Beauty Skin Perfector

FOUNDATION
Maia's Mineral Galaxy Mineral Cream Foundation
Gourmet Body Treats Liquid Mineral Foundation
Delizioso Skincare Dual Active Foundation
Vapour Organic Beauty Atmosphere Foundation
Lauren Brooke Cosmetiques Creme Foundation

STIPPLING BRUSH
MAC 187 Duo Fibre Face Brush
Real Techniques Stippling Brush

CONCEALER
Crush Groove Cosmetics Concealer Puddin'
Delizioso Skincare Organic Pigmented Concealer
Zosimos Botanicals Vegan Concealer
Maia's Mineral Galaxy Concealer Stick
RMS Beauty Un Cover Up
Lauren Brooke Cosmetiques Creme Concealer
Au Naturale Cosmetics Creme Concealer

Vapour Organic Beauty Illusionist Concealer
Miessence Concealer

FINISHING POWDER
Gourmet Body Treats Raw Finishing Powder
Zosimos Botanicals Pristine Finishing Powder
Lauren Brooke Cosmetiques Finishing Powder

FINISHING POWER BRUSH
Ecotools Retractable Kabuki
E.L.F. Studio Powder Brush
It Cosmetics Heavenly Luxe Powder Brush
EcoTools Bamboo Powder Brush
Sonia Kashuk Powder Brush
Everyday Minerals Long handled Kabuki
Alison Raffaele Kabuki Powder Brush
Trish McEvoy Powder Brush #5
Lumiere Kabuki Brush
Sephora Professional Mineral Powder Brush #45
Urban Decay Powder Brush
Real Techniques Expert Face Brush

FACIAL SPRAY
Avène Thermal Spring Water
La Roche-Posay Thermal Spring Water
Releve' Organic Skincare Bamboo Mist
Lauren Brooke Cosmetiques Revitalizing Hydration Tonique

BRONZER
Gourmet Body Treats Hydrating Liquid Bronze
Vapour Organic Beauty Solar Translucent Bronzer
100% Pure Cocoa Pigmented Bronzer
Zosimos Botanicals Butternut Bronzer

BRONZER BRUSH
MAC 167SH Face Blender Brush
Ecotools Bamboo Bronzer Brush
Sephora Professionnel Platinum Bronzer Brush #48

ILLUMINATOR
Vapour Organic Beauty Trick Stick Highlighter Star
Ilia Beauty Illuminator Polka Dots Moonbeams
100% Pure Fruit Pigmented Pink Champagne Luminescent Powder
RMS Beauty Living Luminizer

EYE MAKEUP

The perfect application of eye makeup requires precise detail. Therefore, eye makeup is best used in a stick form so that it can be precisely applied. Eye shadow in the form of a jumbo stick does not leave messy loose powder all over the face. A creamy waterproof eye shadow stick works well for the crease and eyelids since it is long lasting.

Fashion dolls have eye makeup that is designed to make the eyes look larger. To create the appearance of large eyes start by applying white eye shadow on your eyelids. Then define your eyes with a very thin line of black, liquid eyeliner on your top lash line and brown eyeliner on your bottom lash line. Applying black eyeliner all the way around the eyes can make the eyes appear smaller in some women. Apply a dark brown or black in your eye crease with an eye shadow stick. Then apply a neutral or flesh toned eye shadow on your brown bone with an eye shadow stick. The brow bone is the best place to experiment with other eye shadow colors if you so decide. Finally, apply a black lengthening and thickening mascara on your top lashes, and brown mascara on your bottom lashes.

Christian Dior DiorShow Maximizer Lash Plumping Serum is a mascara primer to be applied before putting on mascara. It separates lashes, adds volume, and prevents mascara from clumping.

Shiseido Nourishing Mascara Base is a mascara primer to be applied before putting on mascara. It lengthens, keeps lashes curled, and prevents mascara from clumping.

Etude House Dr. Mascara Fixer for Perfect Lash is a mascara primer to be applied before putting on mascara. It keeps lashes curled, and prevents mascara from smudging. It is somewhat difficult to remove.

Kiko Cosmetics Lengthening Top Coat, available in Europe, is a topcoat to be applied after mascara. It separates and lengthens lashes providing a lash-extension effect.

Overall Beauty Magic Lash Eyelash Enhancer is a topcoat to be applied after mascara. It lengthens and thickens lashes, but needs to be applied properly to work well.

Clarins Double Fix is a topcoat to be applied after putting on mascara. It lets you turn your favorite mascara into waterproof, long lasting mascara. It is somewhat difficult to remove, and is best used for special occasions or when water resistance for mascara is required.

Very thick and long eyelashes as seen on fashion dolls are extremely feminine. Most fashion dolls only have eight or nine extremely thick and long eyelashes. Mascara is fine for everyday wear but false eyelashes create impact for special occasions. To create the dramatically feminine doll eyelash effect, you can use "spike false eyelashes" that are made up of extremely thick and long false eyelashes.

EYEBROW PENCIL
Zosimos Botanicals Brow Pencil
My Earth Natural Cosmetics Eyebrow Pencil
Boots No7 Beautiful Brows Pencil
Sephora Collection Retractable Brow Pencil
Wet 'n' Wild Color Icon Brow & Eye Liner

EYESHADOW PRIMER
Zosimos Botanicals Concealer
Delizioso Skincare Pure Primer
Maia's Mineral Galaxy Liquid Primer

EYELID WHITE SHADOW
Delizioso Skincare Treasure Pearl
Lauren Brooke Cosmetiques Creme Eyeshadow White Satin
Zosimos Botanicals White Hilite Eye Shadow Stick
Au Naturale Cosmetics Creme Eye Shadow in White Quartz
100% Pure Fruit Pigmented Halo Satin Eye Shadow
Sephora Collection Jumbo Liner 12HR Wear Waterproof White

EYE CREASE SHADOW
Delizioso Skincare Cocoa Bean Eyeliner
Lauren Brooke Cosmetiques Creme Eyeshadow Dark Cocoa
Gourmet Body Treats Vegan Eye Pencil Dark Brown
Zosimos Botanicals Black Eye Shadow Stick
Au Naturale Cosmetics Creme Eye Shadow in Saddle
100% Pure Fruit Pigmented Cream Stick Eye Liner Chocolate
Sephora Collection Jumbo Liner 12HR Wear Waterproof Dark Brown

BROW BONE SHADOW
Delizioso Skincare Bronze Sunlight Creamstick Eyeshadow
Lauren Brooke Cosmetiques Creme Eyeshadow Dulce De Leche
Vapour Organic Beauty Mesmerize Eye Color Flash or Charm
Au Naturale Cosmetics Creme Eye Shadow in Coffee or Roseate
Gourmet Body Treats Vegan Eye Pencil Light Brown
100% Pure Fruit Pigmented Bora Bora Satin Eye Shadow
Sephora Collection Jumbo Liner 12HR Wear Waterproof Beige

UPPER EYE LID LIQUID BLACK EYELINER
Gourmet Body Treats Liquid Eye Liner Black
100% Pure Creamy Liquid Eye Liner Black Tea
Jane Iredale Liquid Eye Liner Black
Sephora Collection Nano Eyeliner Midnight Black

LOWER EYE LID BROWN EYELINER
Delizioso Skincare Cocoa Bean Eyeliner
Gourmet Body Treats Vegan Eye Pencil Dark Brown
Zosimos Botanicals Branch Eye Pencil
Sephora Collection Flashy Liner Waterproof Flashy Ultra Brown

MASCARA PRIMER / TOPCOAT
Christian Dior DiorShow Maximizer Lash Plumping Serum
Shiseido Nourishing Mascara Base
Etude House Dr. Mascara Fixer For Perfect Lash
Kiko Cosmetics Lengthening Top Coat
Overall Beauty Magic Lash Eyelash Enhancer
Clarins Double Fix

UPPER LASHES BLACK MASCARA
Delizioso Skincare Black Diamond Nourishing Mascara
Boots Natural Collection Lash Length Mascara Black
Skinfood Almond Volume King Mascara

100% Pure Fruit Pigmented Mascara Black Tea
Lumene True Natural Volume Mascara Black
Korres Provitamin B5 & Rice Bran Mascara
Ecco Bella FlowerColor Natural Mascara

LOWER LASHES BROWN MASCARA
Jane Iredale PureLash Lengthening Mascara Agate Brown
Boots Natural Collection Water Guard Mascara Brown
Lumene True Natural Volume Mascara Brown
Sephora Collection Full Action Extreme Effect Mascara Brown
100% Pure Fruit Pigmented Mascara Dark Chocolate

FALSE UPPER EYELASHES
NYX Fabulous Lashes Eyelashes Pair EL 129 Extreme Measures
Ardell Fashion Lashes 134 Black
Elegant Lashes M075 Mystic Lash
Ardell Fright Night Spyder Woman Lash

EYELASH ADHESIVE
Duo Professional Eyelash Adhesive
Novalash Platinum Bond Lash Adhesive
MAC Lash Adhesive

BLUSH

Blush should be the least heavily applied makeup since heavy blush application is the number one complaint of many men. American actress Chloe Sevigny said, "I find most men don't like a lot of makeup." This applies especially to blush. Examine the fashion doll and notice that blush is barely visible and flesh toned.

Select a flesh toned blush one to three shades darker than your natural skin color. Peach blush color looks the most natural. Blush is best used in a cheek tint or pot rouge so that is can be blended seamlessly into the skin to give a completely sheer and natural look that lasts for hours. Use a duo fiber blush to apply and blend the blush into the cheeks. If you are using a stick blush, then apply on the cheeks and blend the blush into the cheeks with clean fingers.

FLESH TONED BLUSH
100% Pure Peach Glow Lip and Cheek Tint
Gourmet Body Treats Whipped Mousse Blush Apricot
Revolution Organics Freedom Glow Beauty Balm Sunkissed
Au Naturale Cosmetics Lip & Cheek Tint in Vermilion
Zosimos Botanicals Dahlia Lip & Cheek Tint
Crush Groove Cosmetics Cream Chic Mineral Blush
RMS Beauty Lip2Cheek Smile
Vapour Organic Beauty Aura Multi-Use Blush Spark
Ilia Beauty Multi-Stick I Put a Spell on You

BLUSH BRUSH
Too Faced Kabuki Brush
HIRO #42 Travel Powder Kabuki Brush
MAC 188 Duo Fibre Face Brush
Jane Iredale Handi Brush
Shu Uemura Natural 18 Goat Brush
EcoTools Bamboo Blush Brush
Sonia Kashuk Synthetic Flat Top Multipurpose Brush
E.L.F. Studio Blush Brush

LIP MAKEUP

Although the ideal eye and blush color is fairly set (neutral and flesh tones), a woman can have more fun and play around with different natural-looking lip colors and shades such red, pink, peach, and purple.

Before putting on lip color, apply a silicone-based (dimethicone) lip color primer to make the lips appear very smooth and for lip color to stay on better. A lip color primer leads to perfect lipstick application.

Lip balm should ideally consist of simple and healthy ingredients such as shea butter and coconut oil. Lip balm should be without any fragrance, even essential oils, which can be irritating to the lips.

Cosmesis Lip Plumper is a lip plumping treatment to be used three times per day. *Gourmet Body Treats* Glossy Lip Plumper and *Nutra Luxe* Luscious Lip Plumper add subtle volume and gloss to the lips and can be worn instead of lipstick.

LIP COLOR PRIMER
Citrix CRS 15% Cell Rejuvenation Serum
JaDora Cosmetics Skin Primer

LIP LINER
Gourmet Body Treats Vegan Lip Liner Neutral
Afterglow Cosmetics Organic Pencil Lip Liner Bliss
Au Naturale Cosmetics Lip Liner
Zosimos Botanicals Lip Liner Pencils
Sephora Collection Nano Lip Liner

LIP GLOSS
Maia's Mineral Galaxy Transparent Lip Gloss
Gourmet Body Treats Gourmet Lip Gloss
Intelligent Nutrients Gloss Clear Frosting
Vapour Organic Beauty Elixir Lip Gloss Hush

RED LIP COLOR
Gourmet Body Treats Organic Lip Tint
100% Pure Cosmetics Fruit Pigmented Lip Glaze Fruit Punch
Zosimos Botanicals Raspberry Lip Gloss
Delizioso Skincare Red Mango
Maia's Mineral Galaxy Lipstick Precious
Vapour Organic Beauty Siren Lipstick Ravish

Au Naturale Cosmetics Lip Gloss in Dusty Crimson
Kjaer Weis Lip Tint Goddess
Terra Firma Cosmetics Longevity Lip Stain Berry

PINK LIP COLOR
Vapour Organic Beauty Elixir Lip Gloss Twinkle
Lily Lolo Scandalips Lip Gloss
Delizioso Skincare 100% Luxury Natural Lipstick Orchid Petals
Maia's Mineral Galaxy Lipstick Rose Quartz
100% Pure Fruit Pigmented Perfect Naked Mauve Creamstick
Gourmet Body Treats Hydrating Vegan Lipstick Hot Shot
Zosimos Botanicals Peony Lipstick
Afterglow Cosmetics Organic Lip Love Lipstick Wink
Au Naturale Cosmetics Lip & Cheek Tint in Parisian Pink
Maia's Mineral Galaxy Lipstick Rose Quartz
RMS Beauty Lip Shine Sublime
Kjaer Weis Lip Tint Bliss Full
Terra Firma Cosmetics Longevity Lip Stain Pomegranate

PEACH LIP COLOR
Zosimos Botanicals Coral Lipstick
100% Pure Fruit Pigmented Lip Glaze Peach
Lily Lolo Peachy Keen Lip Gloss
Delizioso Skincare 100% Luxury Natural Lipstick Grapefruit
Vapour Organic Beauty Siren Lipstick Saucy
Jane Iredale PureMoist LipColour Kelly
Edward Bess Ultra Slick Lipstick Secret Desire
Kjaer Weis Lip Tint Sweetness
Terra Firma Cosmetics Longevity Lip Stain Bloom

PURPLE LIP COLOR
Zosimos Botanicals Lilac Lipstick
Delizioso Skincare 100% Luxury Natural Lipstick Grape
Maia's Mineral Galaxy Lipstick French Rose
Afterglow Cosmetics Organic Lip Love Lipstick Mystic
Au Naturale Cosmetics Creme Lipstick in Plumeria
Korres Mango Butter Lipstick in Natural Purple
Terra Firma Cosmetics Longevity Lip Stain Vineyard

LIP BRUSH
MAC #318 Retractable Lip Brush
Shu Uemura Kolinsky Portable Extra Lip Brush
Cargo Covered Lip Brush
Urban Decay Lip Brush
Anna Sui Covered Lip Brush
Sonia Kashuk Covered Lip Brush
Bloom Aluminum Lip Brush
Stila #6 Lip Brush
Maybelline Retractable Lip Brush

LIP BALM

Cococare 100% Cocoa Butter The Yellow Stick
Avalon Organics Un-petroleum Lip Balm
Badger Cocoa Butter Lip Balm
Lip Vitamins Lip Balm
Dr. Bronner's Magic Organic Naked Lip Balm
Mode De Vie Karite Lips Shea Butter Lip Balm
Softlips Pure Organic Lip Conditioner Acai Berry
RMS Beauty Lip and Skin Balm Simply Vanilla
Boots Botanics Organic Lip Balm
Alverde Calendula Lip Balm
By Valenti Guava & Watermelon Vegan Lip Balm
Eco Lips Pure & Simple Coconut
eos Lip Balm Sphere
Face Naturals Organic Creme Brulee Lip Balm
Terressentials 100% Organic White Chocolate Lip Protector
Golden Naturals Moisturizing Lip Balm with Kokum Butter
Buddha Nose Certified Organic Lip Balm

LIP PLUMER

Cosmesis Lip Plumper
Gourmet Body Treats Glossy Lip Plumper
Nutra Luxe Luscious Lip Plumper

MAKEUP TOOLS

It is best to use a cosmetic spatula when mixing or measuring beauty products to keep them bacteria-free. It is important to clean your makeup brushes regularly because they collect bacteria. Ideally, you should clean them once per week, or once every two weeks. Many experts say that once a month is fine. Add makeup brush cleaner to one glass of warm water and then dip the brushes into the water. Then, rinse, blot the brush with a clean towel, and use a blow dryer or leave to dry.

The easiest method of removing makeup is to buy wet makeup remover pads or swabs to wipe off makeup. You can also use organic coconut oil mixed with castor oil or olive oil with cosmetic cotton pads.

EYEBROWS

Tweezerman Mini Slant Tweezers
Tweezerman Brow Scissors
Ardell Brow Perfection Stencils

MAKEUP PENCIL SHARPENER

Urban Decay Grindhouse Sharpener
Lancome 2 In 1 Sharpener

COSMETIC SPATULA

Graftobian Flat Mixing Spatula

Zosimos Botanicals Medium White Spatula

MAKEUP BRUSH CLEANSER
Zosimos Botanicals Brush Cleaner
Jane Iredale Botanical Brush Cleaner
Paula Dorf Brush Out Brush Cleaner
Lumene Cosmetic Brush Cleaner
Cinema Secrets Brush Cleaner

MAKEUP REMOVER
Zosimos Botanicals Unscented Makeup Remover Pads
Ava Anderson Non-Toxic Eye Make Up Remover Pads
Jane Iredale Dot the i Makeup Remover Swabs
Almay Gently Clean Non-Oily Face Makeup Remover Pads
Johnson & Johnson Gentle Eye Makeup Remover Pads
DHC Cleansing Oil

Chapter 3: Skin

Beauty is but a flower, which wrinkles will devour.
- Thomas Nashe, English poet

For all skin care products, the general holistic rule is that if it can't be eaten then it shouldn't be applied on the skin. Ingredients should be vitamins, minerals, organic plant or food extracts. If you don't understand what the ingredient is than most likely it is toxic. Many preservatives and chemicals are very harmful to general health. The two most common health-hazardous ingredients are sodium lauryl sulfate (SLS) and propylene glycol. You may also want to avoid fragrance, alcohol, and glycerin in skin care products. Fragrance is a major skin irritant. Many women have found that overtime both glycerin and alcohol have led to dehydrated skin that constantly needs moisturizing.

Whether homemade or commercially bought, it is best to keep all skin products in a wine chiller to keep them as fresh and effective as possible.

The best place to find and purchase the selected skin care products in this chapter is on www.amazon.com, www.skinstore.com, www.dermstore.com, www.vitacost.com, www.iherb.com, or brand websites.

TOP SKIN CARE BRANDS
IMAGE Skincare
www.imageskincare.com

ARCONA
www.arcona.com

DeVita
www.devitaskincare.com

SUNSCREEN

Sunscreen should be treated like the most important beauty product and youth preserver. Zinc oxide is a physical sunscreen that is the most effective active sunscreen ingredient available. It is a mineral that sits on the skin, absorbing and scattering damaging UVA, UVB, and even UVC rays. Zinc oxide sunscreen should be free of nanoparticles (larger than 100 nanometers), to prevent deep absorption of zinc oxide into the skin.

Sunscreen should be unscented, since fragrance can be irritating to the skin. Sunscreen is also more comfortable to wear if it is non-greasy, so that clothing and sand doesn't attach to the skin. A stick form of sunscreen tends to be the least greasy and is suitable to wear on the face, while a cream or aerosol spray form can be used on the body. Aerosol spray sunscreen is extremely fast and easy to put on, but be very careful not to inhale the fumes. Zinc oxide sunscreen should be reapplied every two hours for optimal protection against the sun.

Beta-carotene supplementation helps protect against sunburn. However, a minimum of 10 weeks of supplementation is required before protection is provided. Beta-carotene taken at a dose of 30 milligrams per day helps prevent and repair photoaging.

Polypodium leucotomos extract and astaxanthin are two powerful natural UV protectors. *Raintree Nutrition* Calaguala Capsules contains polypodium leucotomos extract, which is a natural fern extract that protects the skin from sun damage and photoaging. It also slows the absorption of harmful UV rays and prevents DNA damage.

ZINC OXIDE FACE SUNSCREEN
Elemental Herbs Sunstick Zinc Sunscreen Unscented SPF 30
Raw Elements USA Eco Stick SPF 30+
Purple Prairie Botanicals SunStick Mineral Stick SPF 30
IMAGE Skincare Prevention+ Daily Ultimate Protection SPF 50

ZINC OXIDE LIP SUNSCREEN
BurnOut Lip Balm Natural Coconut SPF 32
Devita Lip Volumizer SPF 15
Loving Naturals Clear Lips SPF 30+
Badger Unscented Lip Balm SPF 15
Purple Prairie Botanicals SunStuff Lip Balm SPF 30

ZINC OXIDE BODY SUNSCREEN
All Terrain TerraSport Sunscreen Spray SPF 30
IMAGE Skincare Prevention+ Daily Hydrating SPF 30
Replenix Ultra Sheer Physical Sunscreen Spray SPF 50
Marie Veronique Organics Kid Safe Screen SPF 25
Goddess Garden Organics Sunny Body Organic Sunscreen Continuous Spray
EltaMD UV Aero Broad-Spectrum SPF 45
Poofy Organics The Sunscreen SPF 30
Pratima Skin Care Neem Rose Body Sunscreen SPF 30
Loving Naturals Clear Face Sunscreen SPF 30+
Releve' Organic Skincare Sun-Lite SPF 20

Karen's Botanicals Simple Sun Block Unscented SPF 30
Kabana Skin Care Green Screen D Organic SPF 35
Erbaviva Natural Sunscreen SPF 30
Osmosis Shelter SPF 30
Thinksport Livestrong Sunscreen SPF 50+
BurnOut Eco-Sensitive Sunscreen SPF 30
Devita Solar Body Block SPF 30+
MyChelle Replenishing Solar Defense SPF 30

SUNSCREEN PILL
Now Foods Beta Carotene
Now Foods Astaxanthin
Raintree Nutrition Calaguala Capsules

FACIAL PRODUCTS

The most powerful tools for preventing and reversing skin aging, besides zinc oxide sunscreen, are tretinoin and vitamin C serum. Collagen degradation doesn't generally start until the mid-twenties, so it's best to start using tretinoin and vitamin C serum in one's mid-twenties.

To start using tretinoin, use the 0.025% strength for a few months. Apply once every three days for the first one or two weeks. After the skin adjusts to the product, use it up to once every two nights for another few weeks. Then, use it every other night for another week and then nightly. You can eventually graduate to the 0.05% strength and use it every day for one full year. After one year, you can graduate to the 0.1% strength and use it two to four times per week. Many dermatologists advice that 2-3 times a week is plenty. Some women choose to use it only once a week. Always wear sunscreen during the day, and apply tretinoin at night before bed since tretinoin makes your skin more sensitive to the sun.

The use of tretinoin can leave the skin dry. Therefore a moisturizer can be applied 1 hour after tretinoin application. You must wait an hour after applying tretinoin to apply moisturizer so you do not diminish the effects of the tretinoin. The best antiaging moisturizer contains both peptides and ceramides. Ceramides help keep moisture in the skin while peptides increase collagen production. You can also add lactic acid to the moisturizer to treat very dry skin. Add 2.5 teaspoons of 88% lactic acid to two teaspoons of moisturizer. You can buy 88% lactic acid from www.lotioncrafter.com or www.skinessentialactives.com.

There are a few options to choose from on days that tretinoin is not used. Glycolic acid serum or kinetin/NAG/niacinamide serum is a great addition to an antiaging skin care regimen and can be used on days when tretinoin is not used. Idebenone is another antiaging ingredient that can be used in place of the kinetin in the NAG/niacinamide serum. Botox gel is effective for women 35 and under who do not need Botox yet, but want to prevent wrinkles from forming.

A cleanser that contains alpha hydroxy acids (AHA) is a good way to exfoliate dead skin cells and reverse skin aging. Another effective method of exfoliating the skin is to use chemical peels. Doing chemical peels at home is convenient and cost effective. Each chemical peel is categorized by the concentration and the resulting depth of the peel on the skin, which can range from superficial (also known as micro or light peels) to medium, or deep peels. Results are closely linked to the depth of peel performed. Superficial peels (AHA or BHA) offer less dramatic improvement than medium or deep peels (Jessner's or TCA). However, several mild- to medium-depth peels can achieve similar results to one deep-peel treatment, with less post-procedure risk and a shorter recovery time.

Pumpkin peels at 30% can be used every week and are well tolerated by sensitive skin. They contain a high concentration of beta-carotene and vitamins A and C, which encourage the production of collagen and elastin. Pumpkin also possesses nutrients like zinc and potassium that nourish the skin, while natural AHAs and enzymes exfoliate.

Mandelic acid is a gentle acid that exfoliates the skin with very little topical discomfort and can be used at 25% every week. It is helpful for inhibiting the formation of brown spots and hyperpigmentation. It helps treat melasma, sun damage, large pores, wrinkles, and dull and sallow skin.

Glycolic acid stimulates collagen growth more effectively than any of the other chemical peels. Its small molecule allows it to slip beneath the epidermis to reach the collagen fibers below. Glycolic acid peels are best used every month at 70% to prevent and reverse skin aging. Begin by using 30% and work your way up slowly to using a 70% glycolic acid peel.

Trichloroacetic acid (TCA) peels can be done at home or by a dermatologist and are very effective at removing skin imperfections such as lines, wrinkles, hyperpigmentation, sun damage, lip lines, and age spots. It is excellent for spot peeling of specific areas. Start at 12.5% for three months, moved up to 20% for six months, and then move up to 30%. Do not go higher than 30% for a TCA peel. You can perform one TCA peel every five weeks until skin imperfections fade and then perform a TCA peel once a year.

Sleeping on a "beauty pillow" will help prevent wrinkles. While sleeping on the specially designed pillow, your head gently hangs off the side of the pillow, preventing your face from pressing into the pillow and developing wrinkles.

At-home electronic devices such as the microneedle roller, LED light therapy, microcurrent, or ultrasonic waves have been shown to be effective for many women in reducing the signs of skin aging and are a good addition to any anti-aging routine.

To begin using a microneedle roller, start with a 0.5mm, twice a week. Within a few months you can try using a 1.5mm, once every 3 weeks. You can use a 2.0mm on skin scars, every 5 weeks. Many women apply a serum with copper peptides and hyaluronic acid during each microneedle roller session.

Specific supplements and superfoods are very beneficial for preventing skin aging. Vitamin C, Pycnogenol, evening primrose oil, MSM, carnosine, milk thistle, astaxanthin, pearl powder, and certain Chinese remedies have helped many women look younger for longer.

FACIAL CLEANSER

Goat Milk Stuff Goat Milk Soap Purity
Alabu Moisturizing Goat Milk Soap
Creamery Creek Unscented Goat Milk Soap
Ajara Ayurvedic Beauty Rosacea Facial Cleanser
Frownies pH Balanced Complexion Wash
Beauty Without Cruelty Facial Cleanser 3% AHA Complex
ARCONA Berry Fruit Bar
100% Pure Skin Brightening Facial Cleansing

VITAMIN C SERUM

Forever Young Store Vitamin C Serum (25%)
Biopeutic Vitamin C + Fullerenes Whitening Serum (25%)
IMAGE Skincare Vital C Hydrating A C & E Serum (20%)
NuFountain Fresh Cosmetics C20 Vitamin C Serum (20%)
ARCONA Youth Serum (20%)
Cellex-C Advanced C-Serum (17.5%)
DeVita Topical Vitamin C Serum (17%)
Glo Professional Ultra Vitamin C (15%)
Nutra-Lift Maximum C Plus Serum
Golden Naturals Collagen Buster Serum
Destiny Boutique Vitamin C Serum
Marie Veronique Organics Pacific Topical Vitamin C Treatment

TRETINOIN

Retin-A Gel (0.025%-0.1%)
Skin Peel Shop Retinoic Acid Cream (0.1%)

RETINOL/ROSEHIP SERUM

Life Flo Health Retinol A 1%
ARCONA Vitamin A Complex
IMAGE Skincare Ageless Total Retinol A Crème
Glo Professional Tretinol 0.5%
Be Natural Organics Bio-Recovery Face Serum
Korres Rose Hips Face Serum
Akin Pure Alchemy Cellular Radiance Serum
Bare Organics Organic Facial Serum Unscented

EYE TREATMENT

Cellex-C Advanced-C Eye Toning Gel
ARCONA Night Worker
Dr. Alkaitis Organic Eye Crème
JabaLabs Milexin MD
Reviva Labs Under-Eye Dark Circle Serum
Glo Professional 7.5% Vitamin C Eye Gel
Watts Beauty Vanish Extreme Under Eye Cream
Releve' Organic Skincare Exhilar-Eyes Eye Renewal Cream
HollyBeth's Natural Luxury Eye Cream
Glam-Nation Organic Eye Cream
Herbaliz Eye Cream

Cosmesis Dark Circle & Puffiness Remover Serum
Be Natural Organics Eye Repair Night Serum
Nature's Pharma Eye Serum Oil
Immunocologie Eye Repair Treatment Crème
University Medical Wrinkle MD Eye

MOISTURIZER
IMAGE Skincare Vital C Hydrating Anti Aging Serum
IMAGE Skincare The Max Serum
Sweet Wheat Sweet Skin Botanical Moisturizing Cream
Subversive Apothecary Anti-aging Serum
Ecco Bella Night Rebuilder Cream
Perlage Fortifying Rejuvenation Treatment
Immunocologie Treatment Creme
Skin Perfection Expression Line Deep Wrinkle Serum
Sevani Beauty Phyto-Peptide Firming Face Cream
Devita Shea Butter Brulée
Perfect Organics Perfection Cream
Releve' Organic Skincare Luxotic Organic Face Moisturizer

GLYCOLIC ACID SERUM
IMAGE Skincare Ageless Total Anti Aging Serum
Devita High Performance Glycolic Acid Blend Serum
Reviva Labs 10% Glycolic Acid Cream
Earth Science Active Age Defense Hydroxy Acid Night Rejuvenator
Glo Professional Renew Serum
Mad Hippie Skin Care Products Exfoliating Serum

FRUIT ENZYME MASK
Lily Organics Rejuvenating Enzyme Mask
Bryce Organics Jamaican Papaya Enzyme Facial Peel
Happy Pumpkin Enzyme Peel
Glo Professional Pumpkin Enzyme Scrub
Releve' Organic Skincare Nutri-Zyme Organic Peel
Earth Science Gentle Skin Peel Papaya-Glycolic
Abra Therapeutics Alpha Enzyme Peel

BOTOX GEL
Skin Peel Shop Botox Gel

LIGHTENING
Abella Enliten Skin Bleaching Cream
PCA pHaze 13 Pigment Gel
Ultraquin Cream 4%
ARCONA Lightening Drops

PROBLEM SKIN CARE
Lumina Health Cell Food Oxygenating Skin Care Oxygen Gel
IMAGE Skincare Clear Cell Medicated Acne Lotion
ARCONA AM Acne Lotion
ARCONA Night Breeze

EXFOLIATING PEELS
iskyn pro Pumpkin Peel
Forever Young 20% Mandelic Malic Acid Peel
Makeup Artists Choice 25% Mandelic Acid Peel
Makeup Artists Choice 15% Salicylic Acid
Skin Obsession 85% Lactic Acid Peel
Skin Obsession Glycolic Acid Peel
Skin Obsession Jessner's Chemical Peel
Skin Peel Shop Retinoic Acid Solution
Skin Obsession TCA Chemical Peel

MICROFIBER CLOTH
Buf-Puf Facial Sponge
NCN Pro Microfiber Cleansing Cloth

SKIN CARE DEVICES
Cynergy Derma Roller
LightStim LED Light Therapy
NuFace Microcurrent Device
Tua tre'nd Microcurrent Device
SkinDream TITANIUM Ultrasonic Device
DermaWand Radio Frequency
Vaculifter Skin and Facial Massage Therapy
Safetox Beauty
JeNu Active-Youth Skincare System

MICROCURRENT GALVANIC GEL
Rankine's Remedies Galvanic Treatment System

FACIAL EXERCISE
FlexEffect Facialbuilding
Senta Maria Rungé Face Lifting By Exercise
The Eigard Method

BEAUTY PILLOW
Vasseur Skincare International Beauty Pillow
Arc4life Cervical Linear Traction Neck Pillow

SKIN SUPPLEMENTS
Now Foods Tru-C BioComplex
Healthy Origins Pycnogenol
Now Foods Super Primrose
Doctor's Best MSM
Now Foods L-Carnosine
Now Foods Silymarin Milk Thistle Extract 2X
Healthy Origins Astaxanthin
Dragon Herbs Pearl Powder
Dragon Herbs 8 Immortals

BODY PRODUCTS

The most publicly exposed areas of the body can receive the same skin care routine as the face. Tretinoin, serums, moisturizers, masks, peels, and electronic devices can be used on the hands, arms, shoulders, neck, and below the neck. The rest of the body such as the legs, stomach, breasts, and back can be treated with glycolic acid or lactic acid lotion at night and vitamin C cream in the morning along with zinc oxide sunscreen.

Lactic acid lotion is very beneficial for relieving and preventing dry skin. Lactic acid lotion is made in small batches since it expires quickly. To make lactic acid lotion, add 2.5 teaspoons of 88% lactic acid to two teaspoons of any lotion. The best body lotion contains both peptides and ceramides. Ceramides help keep moisture in the skin while peptides increase collagen production.

Natural oils can replace the use of commercially prepared moisturizers and can reverse many skin problems. They are also useful for body massages performed at spas. You can use grape seed oil, squalene oil, rose hip seed oil, jojoba oil, borage seed oil, avocado oil, or sea buckthorn oil.

Compression stocking increase circulation within the legs which brings much-needed nutrients and oxygenated blood into the legs and feet. Compression therapy can regenerate damaged tissues. Women suffering from conditions such as varicose veins, arthritis, leg ulcers and lymphoedema can all benefit from the healing properties of compression.

Feet need special skin care since the bottom of the feet tends to get very rough and dry. Apply a lactic acid lotion and special "moisturizing socks" every night before bed. Mafura butter is great for applying to the feet during the daytime since it's not greasy and is very emollient.

BODY WASH
Elemis Skin Nourishing Shower Cream
Eminence Organics Naseberry Cranberry Yogurt Body Wash
Frownies pH Balanced Complexion Wash
Kahina Giving Beauty Facial Cleanser
IMAGE Skincare Body Spa Body Exfoliating Scrub

BODY DAY LOTION
IMAGE Skincare Vital C Hydrating Repair Creme
Cellex-C Advanced C Skin Tightening Cream
Reviva Labs Alpha Lipoic Acid Vitamin C Ester & DMAE Cream
Avalon Organics Vitamin C Renewal Cream

BODY NIGHT LOTION
Cellex-C Betaplex New Complexion Cream
IMAGE Skincare Body Spa Rejuvenating Body Lotion
ARCONA Pumpkin Body Lotion 10 Percent
Reviva Labs Glycolic Acid Cream (5%-10%)

MASSAGE LOTION / OIL
Primavera Grapeseed Oil
IQ Natural 100% Pure Squalene
Primavera Rose Hip Oil
Primavera Jojoba Oil
Raw Gaia Organic Borage Seed Oil
Life Flo Health Pure Avocado Oil
Life Flo Health Pure Sea Buckthorn Oil
Marula The Leakey Collection
Nature Certified Organic Oil Blend
Earth Mama Angel Baby Natural Stretch Oil
Jason Natural Vitamin E 5,000 I.U. Pure Natural Skin Oil
Global Healing Center O2-Zap
ARCONA Green Tea Lotion
Releve' Organic Skincare Organic Body Lotion
Crush Groove Cosmetics Creme de Nude Head-to-Toe Body Butter
Temptations Bath n' Body Body Icing

LEG COMPRESSION
RejuvaHealth Compression Stockings

FOOT MOISTURIZER
Earth Therapeutics TheraSoft Moisturizing Socks
Airplus Aloe Infused Ultra Moisturizing Socks
MediPeds Moisturizing Socks with Aloe Vera
Of A Simple Nature Mafura Butter
Cebra Ethical Skincare Mafura Butter
Rain Africa Macadamia Mafura Body Butter

DEODORANT
Nourish Fresh Stick Deodorant Organic Wild Greens
Crystal Body Deodorant Roll-On
Naturally Fresh Deodorant Crystal Mini Roll On
Kabana Naturally Effective Deodorant
Aura Cacia Aromatherapy Roll-On Stick
Crystalux Crystal Stick Deodorant
Lafe's Natural BodyCare Deodorant Stick
Face Naturals Himalayan Pink Salt Deodorant Spray
Innocent Oils Himalayan Crystal Body Spray

SUNLESS TANNING
Silk Naturals Self Tanner
Decleor Aroma Sun Express Hydrating Self Tan Spray
Elemental Herbology Sun Kiss Body Hydrator with Self Tan
IMAGE Skincare Body Spa Face and Body Bronzer Crème
Caribbean Solutions Beach Colours Self Tanner
Swissclinical Self-Tanner
Golden Sol Sunless Tanning Mist
Tantrix Organic Tanning Mist
MyChelle Del Sol Sunless Tanner
Vita Liberata Rich Silken Chocolate

Infinity Sun Glow on the Go
Norvell Self-Tanning Aerosol
Sephora Collection Tinted Self-Tanning Body Mist
Bliss A Tan For All Seasons

BODY SHIMMER POWDER
Vapour Organic Beauty Halo Body Spotlight Brilliance
Zosimos Botanicals Cocoa Shimmer Dust
Terra Firma Cosmetics All Over Glow
Bath & Body Works Flawless 24K Shimmer Powder Spray

Chapter 4: Hair

The hair is the richest ornament of women.
- Martin Luther, German monk

Most commercial hair products contain chemicals that slow down hair growth and causes hair shedding. The goal in finding the best hair care products is in finding products with natural ingredients as well as a product that actually works. All selected hair care brands and products in this chapter are natural and help the hair grow faster, thicker, and shiner.

The best place to find and purchase the selected hair care products in this chapter is on: www.amazon.com, or www.iherb.com.

TOP HAIR CARE BRANDS
Aubrey Organics
www.aubrey-organics.com

Avalon Organics
www.avalonorganics.com

Mill Creek
www.millcreekusa.com

Giovanni
www.giovannicosmetics.com

Nature's Gate
www.natures-gate.com

Herbatint
www.herbatintusa.com

HAIR COLORING

The chemicals in hair dyes are extremely damaging to hair and harmful to health. Organic, natural, and non-damaging hair dyes are the best choice.

After coloring the hair, it is important to use a color-protecting or color-enhancing shampoo and conditioner to reduce color fading and keep hair looking vibrant.

PERMANENT HAIR COLOR
Herbatint Permanent Herbal Haircolor Gel
Naturtint Permanent Hair Colorant
Logona Herbal Hair Color
Rainbow Research Henna Hair Color
Light Mountain Natural Hair Color
Sante Herbal Hair Color

COLOR-ENHANCING SHAMPOO
Aquage Sea Extend Silkening Shampoo
Nature's Gate Hair Defense Shampoo
Aveeno Active Naturals Living Color Preserving Shampoo
Giovanni Colorflage Shampoo
Malibu Color Wellness Shampoo
Shikai Natural Color Care Shampoo
Surya Brasil Color Fixation Restorative Shampoo
Save Your Hair Color Safe Shampoo
ABBA Pure Color Protect Shampoo
Hugo Naturals Color Protecting Shampoo

COLOR-ENHANCING CONDITIONER
SeaExtend Silkening Conditioner
Nature's Gate Pomegranate Sunflower Hair Defense Conditioner
Aveeno Active Naturals Living Color Conditioner
Giovanni Colorflage Conditioner
Malibu Color Wellness Conditioner
Shikai Color Reflect Intensive Repair Conditioner
Surya Brasil Color Fixation Restorative Conditioner
Save Your Hair Color Safe Conditioner
ABBA Pure Color Protect Conditioner
Hugo Naturals Color Protecting Conditioner

HAIR LENGTH

To increase the speed of hair growth, look for natural shampoos that contain MSM, amino acids, B vitamins, He Shou Wu, *Russelia equisetiformis*, and *Prunus persica* extract.

One of the best ways to promote faster hair growth is to regularly apply hair-oil treatments. The most effective oils for promoting hair growth are emu oil, amla oil, castor oil, and coconut oil along with the essential oils of rosemary, thyme, lavender, and cedarwood.

During the time you are trying to grow out your hair, it is important to use a leave-in conditioner or some argan oil on the ends of the hair to prevent split ends.

Some women have reported their hair grew faster after taking prenatal vitamins. Prenatal vitamins contain higher concentrations of folic acid, calcium, and iron than regular multivitamins.

Besides prenatal vitamins, other nutrients are beneficial to the hair. Biotin is reported to help hair grow faster, although some women complain that it causes acne. MSM or collagen combined with vitamin C provides sulfur, which is known to promote hair growth. Fish oil contains omega-3 fatty acids, which nourishes the hair follicles.

Herbalists suggest horsetail extract and nettle for stimulating hair growth. Chinese herbalists recommend Fo-Ti, which is also known to prevent hair from becoming gray.

HAIR GROWTH SHAMPOO
Emu Gold Therapeutic Body Care Shampoo and Conditioner
Herbal Glo See More Hair Shampoo
Revita High Performance Hair Growth Stimulating Shampoo
Peter Lamas Chinese Herbs Stimulating Shampoo
Rudy's Emu Oil And Jojoba Oil Shampoo
Longhairlovers Luxe Shampoo
Laid in Montana EMUtrients Shampoo
The Pure Guild Hair Re-Growth Shampoo
Nature's Gate Biotin Strengthening Shampoo

HAIR GROWTH CONDITIONER
Emu Essence Naturals Revitalizing Conditioner
Healthy Hair Plus Emu Oil Conditioner
Herbal Glo See More Hair Conditioner
Revita High Performance Hair Growth Stimulating Conditioner
Peter Lamas Chinese Herbs Stimulating Conditioner
Rudy's Emu Oil And Jojoba Oil Conditioner
Longhairlovers Luxe Conditioner
Laid in Montana EMUtrients Conditioner
The Pure Guild Hair Re-Growth Conditioner

LEAVE-IN CONDITIONER
Giovanni Direct Leave-In Weightless Moisture Conditioner
Madre Labs Leave-In Conditioner
Acure Organics Leave-In Conditioner Argan Oil + Argan Stem Cell
Aura Cacia Organic Argan Oil

HAIR GROWTH SUPPLEMENTS
Viviscal
Rainbow Light Just Once Prenatal One
Now Foods Biotin
Neocell Super Collagen+C
Doctor's Best Best MSM

Natural Factors Omega Factors Wild Alaskan Salmon Oil
Nature's Way Horsetail Grass
Now Foods Nettle Root Extract
Chinese Natural Herbs Alopecia Areata Pill
Active Herb Shou Wu Pian
Dimmak Herbs Han Lian Cao

HAIR SHINE

To get hair it's shiniest use a very hydrating shampoo and conditioner, and rinse with ice-cold water. Then, after hair has dried, use a shine-serum to further smooth out the hair. "Straight hair has great natural shine, because its flat cuticle is highly light-reflective," says New York City salon owner Paul Labrecque. Colorless henna is a treatment that smoothes and seals the hair's cuticle for greater shine.

SHINE SHAMPOO
Giovanni Smooth As Silk Deep Moisture Shampoo
Aubrey Organics Moisturizing Shampoo Honeysuckle Rose
Avalon Organics Deep Moisturizing Shampoo Awapuhi Mango Therapy
Mill Creek Keratin Shampoo Repair Formula
Shikai Henna Gold Highlighting Shampoo
Salon Naturals Sleek & Shiny Shampoo
Madre Labs Moisturizing Shampoo
Nature's Baby Organics Shampoo & Body Wash
Acure Organics Shampoo Moroccan Argan Oil + Argan Stem Cell
NaturOli Extreme Soap Nut Shampoo

SHINE CONDITIONER
Giovanni Smooth As Silk Deeper Moisture Conditioner
Aubrey Organics Moisturizing Conditioner Honeysuckle Rose
Avalon Organics Deep Moisturizing Conditioner Awapuhi Mango Therapy
Mill Creek Keratin Conditioner Repair Formula
Shikai Henna Gold Highlighting Conditioner
Salon Naturals Sleek & Shiny Conditioner
Madre Labs Moisturizing Conditioner
Nature's Baby Organics Conditioner & Detangler
Acure Organics Conditioner Moroccan Argan Oil + Argan Stem Cell
Giovanni 2chic Ultra-Sleek Conditioner Brazilian Keratin & Argan Oil
Desert Essence Conditioner Coconut

SHINE SERUM
Giovanni Frizz Be Gone Super Smoothing Anti-Frizz Hair Serum
Joico K-Pak Protect & Shine Serum
Charles Worthington Shine Silkening Serum
Paves Flawless In the Spotlight Greaseless EO Shine Serum
Garnier Fructis Sleek & Shine Weightless Anti-Frizz Serum
Liquid Keratin Sealing Shine Serum
Hask Pure Shine Polishing Serum
Venetian Blends Shine Serum

Head Organics Hair Shine Serum Anti-Frizz
Salon Naturals Argan Oil Finishing Serum
Face Naturals Shine Serum for Hair

LEAVE-IN CONDITIONER
Giovanni 2chic Ultra Sleek Leave-In Conditioning & Styling Elixir
Kinky-Curly Knot Today Natural Leave in / Detangler
The Jane Carter Solution Revitalizing Leave-In Conditioner
Isvara Organics Leave-In Detangling Spray

COLORLESS HENNA
Rainbow Research Persian Neutral Colorless Conditioner
Morrocco Method Colorless Herbal Conditioner

HAIR VOLUME

Look for organic and natural shampoos with *Russelia equisetiformis*, *Prunus persica* extract, *Swertia japonica* extract, licorice root extract, white peony root extract, rosemary extract, biotin, and panthenol, which help prevent hair loss. Hydrolyzed wheat protein is very effective at adding hair volume to limp hair.

VOLUME SHAMPOO
Avalon Organics Biotin B-Complex Thickening Shampoo
Mill Creek Biotin Shampoo Therapy Formula
Nature's Gate Biotin Strengthening Shampoo
Biotene H-24 Shampoo
Jason Natural Thin to Thick Extra Volume Shampoo
Giovanni Root 66 Max Volume Shampoo
Andalou Naturals Full Volume Shampoo
Beauty Without Cruelty Shampoo Volume Plus
Salon Naturals Volumizing Shampoo
Logona Volume Shampoo Honey Beer

VOLUME CONDITIONER
Avalon Organics Biotin B-Complex Thickening Conditioner
Mill Creek Biotin Conditioner Therapy Formula
Nature's Gate Biotin Conditioner Strengthening
Biotene H-24 Conditioner
Jason Natural Thin to Thick Extra Volume Conditioner
Giovanni Root 66 Max Volume Conditioner
Andalou Naturals Full Volume Conditioner
Beauty Without Cruelty Conditioner Volume Plus
Salon Naturals Volumizing Conditioner

VOLUME SPRAY
Modern Organic Products Lemongrass Lift
Kenra Volume Spray
Simply Organic Volumizing & Thickening Spray
Alterna Bamboo Volume Spray

Giovanni Root 66 Max Volume Directional Root Lifting Spray

EYELASHES & EYEBROWS

Latisse is a prescription solution that produces longer, thicker eye lashes by keeping hairs in their growth phase. The effects of Latisse are not permanent and it can cause eye or eyelid discoloration. *Careprost* and *Lumigan are* the generic versions of *Latisse* and are available from www.alldaychemist.com and www.worldwide-pharmacies.com. *Travatan* (Travoprost) and *Xalatan* (Latanoprost) are ophthalmic solutions for glaucoma to be used as a safe way to grow eyelashes. They are available from www.alldaychemist.com.

EYELASHES & EYEBROWS GROWTH SOLUTION
Latisse / Careprost / Lumigan
Travatan
Xalatan

HAIR TOOLS

A boar-bristle brush is the best choice for brushing. It is excellent at distributing the oils from the scalp to the hair ends and increasing circulation in the scalp, which is important for helping the hair grow.
Perfectly straight hair can be achieved with a good straightening iron. You can also just permanently straighten your hair with Japanese Hair Straightening, also called Thermal Reconditioning or Brazilian Keratin Treatment. Many hair-care professionals prefer tourmaline irons. Wavy hair can be achieved by using a curling iron or hot rollers along with hair spray. You should always use a hair heat-protection treatment before using hair styling irons.

BRUSH
Mason Pearson Pure Bristle Brush
Sonia Kashuk Bristle Hair Brush
Denman Boar Bristle Brush
Frederic Fekkai Travel Brush

HEAT-PROTECTION
John Frieda Frizz-Ease Hair Serum Thermal Protection Formula
Joico K-Pak Thermal Design Foam
Wella High Hair Flat Iron Spray
TIGI S-Factor Flat Iron Shine Spray
Giovanni 2chic Blow Out Styling Mist Brazilian Keratin & Argan Oil

HAIR DRYER
BaByliss Pro Ceramix Xtreme Dryer
Farouk Chi Touch Hair Dryer
Conair Comfort Touch Tourmaline Ceramic Hair Dryer

STRAIGHTENING IRON
Farouk CHI Ceramic Flat Iron
Solano HAI Convertible Flat Iron
GHD Ceramic Flat Iron
Conair i-series Tourmaline Ceramic Flat Iron
Jilbere de Paris Nano Ceramic Ionic Flat Iron

CURLING IRON
Conair Infiniti You Curl No Clamp Curling Iron
Hot Tools Curling Iron Spring Grip
Sultra Bombshell Curling Wand
Pro Beauty Tools Curling Iron
Conair Jumbo Rollers Instant Heat Travel Hairsetter

Chapter 5: Body

Take care of your body. It's the only place you have to live.
- Jim Rohn, American businessman

Waist-to-hip ratio (WHR) and body mass index (BMI) are the two factors that determine the attractiveness of the body. WHR indicates body shape while BMI indicates body size. A woman must take care of her body through diet and exercise if she wants it to be in perfect form. "Revere the body and care for it, for it is a temple," said Indian guru Swami Muktananda.

A wide range of factors, such as biochemical individuality, endocrine/hormonal imbalances, digestive problems, blood sugar fluctuations, candida, food allergies, organ dysfunction, psychological issues, toxic load, can contribute to weight gain or difficulty in weight loss. Therefore, a naturopath can determine and treat the cause of overweight if it remains a problem despite proper diet, supplements, exercise, and cosmetic procedures.

TOP BODY SUPPLEMENT BRANDS
Now Foods
www.nowfoods.com

USP Labs
www.usplabsdirect.com

Natrol
www.natrol.com

Source Naturals
www.sourcenaturals.com

Michael's Naturopathic
www.michaelshealth.com

WAIST-TO-HIP RATIO (WHR)

Before embarking on any program to reduce the size of the waist, it is important to determine the cause of a large mid-section. Once you determine the cause with the help of a naturopath, you can select the right treatment.

Women with high levels of the male sex hormones (androgens) and low levels of estrogen have increased WHR. Lowering androgen levels and increasing estrogen levels will help lower a woman's WHR. Saw palmetto is an antiandrogen and is helpful for lowering androgen levels in the body. Saw palmetto can be combined with goat's rue (*Galega officinalis*) and black cumin seed (*Nigella sativa*), which are known to slim the waist.

Colon detoxification will flush out toxins from the colon and reduce the size of the waist. Colonics are effective for cleansing the colon. The colon can also be cleansed with the herbal combination of cape aloe leaf, rhubarb root, marshmallow root, and triphala churna. Nonaddictive fiber supplements such as flax seeds and oat bran will keep the colon clean.

Cortisol is a hormone that is released in response to stress and tends to deposit fat around the waist. Lowering cortisol levels will reduce the size of the waist for women with stressful lifestyles. Holy basil (*Ocimum sanctum*) is an Indian herb that reduces elevated cortisol levels.

Candida may be a cause of a large waist. Electrodermal screening can detect candida. Candida can be treated with oil of oregano, olive leaf, and grapefruit seed extract. A "candida diet" is also helpful. The candida diet consists of eliminating sugar, carbohydrates, vinegar, mushrooms, cheese, peanuts, and high-sugar fruits for up to one year.

To reduce your waist temporarily, you can wear a corset. Corsets reduce the waist size by two to four inches. A satin or silk corset is the best option if you don't want anyone to see the lumps and bumps typically seen with lace corsets.

Corsets can be selected in either underbust or overbust, depending on preference. Underbust cinch the waist, while overbust cinch the waist as well as supporting and lifting the breasts. The best corsets have steel boning (spring steel, which allows for bend but still gives a great deal of support).

To reduce the size of a number of body parts temporarily, you can wear a seamless full-body shaper. Full-body shapers will slim the thighs, shape the buttocks, and reduce the waist. You can choose extra firm, firm, medium, or light control.

Women that want to permanently reduce their waist size and get the perfect V-shaped waist can consider tightlacing, also called corset training or waist training. The female ribs are flexible, and continuous inward pressure on the ribs will tend to gradually force the bones into a V-shape.

To begin tightlacing, acquire a custom-tailored four or five inches smaller than the waist size. A zipper-closure corset is recommended since it is the fastest to put on. Start by wearing the training corset for a few hours each day and gradually increase the length of time you wear it until you are able to wear it 12 hours a day, every single day. Some women have worn a training corset for up to 23 hours a day. Once you achieve your desired waist size, you can wear the corset for only a few hours per day to maintain your shape.

To enhance the buttocks temporarily, the padded panty will make up for lack of volume. Some padded panties also include hip enhancers and thigh control to increase the size of the hips and reduce the size of the thighs. A butt-lifter panty will lift up the buttocks for women that already have volume but lack firmness.

Many women have reported that taking the herb maca root (*Lepidium meyenii*) internally effectively increased the volume and projection of their buttocks. A strict schedule can be followed to achieve maximum results. Start by taking 1,000 milligrams per day for one week, and add 500 milligrams more every week until you reach week six. At week six you should take a break. At week seven start all over as in week one, taking 1,000 milligrams per day. Instead of following this strict schedule you can simply take 2,200 milligrams per day until achieving the desired results.

Volufiline is a non-hormonal ingredient found in breast growth creams that increases the amount of fat cells in the area to which it is applied leading to permanent volume. You can apply these breast creams to the buttocks.

LOWER ANDROGEN LEVELS
Now Foods Saw Palmetto Berries
Motherlove Goat's Rue
Amazing Herbs Black Seed
Alvita Teas Spearmint Leaf
Celebration Herbals Organic Spearmint Leaf
Michael's Naturopathic Prostate Factors

COLON CLEANSE
Earth's Bounty Oxy-Cleanse Oxygen Colon Conditioner
Mr. Oxygen OxyFlush
Michael's Naturopathic Fiber & More
Uni Key Health Systems Super-GI Cleanse
TerraVita Butternut Bark
Planetary Herbals Triphala
Only Natural Easy Colon Cleaner
Renew Life Organic Bowel Cleanse

CANDIDA CLEANSE
Now Foods Oregano Oil
NutriBiotic Grapefruit Seed Extract
Natural Factors Olive Leaf Extract
Now Foods Betaine HCI
Now Foods Virgin Coconut Oil
Allimax 100% Allicin Powder Capsules
Michael's Naturopathic Paraherbs
Lumina Health Cell Food Oxygen Supplement
Jarrow Formulas Jarro-Dophilus EPS
Dr. Ohhira's Essential Formulas Inc., Probiotics

LOWER CORTISOL
Now Foods Super Cortisol Support
New Chapter Holy Basil
Now Foods Rhodiola
Natural Sources Raw Thyroid
Michael's Naturopathic Thyroid Factors
Enzymatic Therapy Metabolic Advantage Thyroid Formula

TIGHTLACING CORSET
Orchard Corset
Waisted Couture
Corsets Queen
Contour Corsets
Romantasy Exquisite Corsetry

SHAPEWEAR / BODY ENHANCERS
Love My Bubbles
Feel Foxy
Hour Glass Angel
Silicone Body
Lauren Silva
Body Shapers Unlimited
Beauty Lies Beneath
ResultWear

BUTTOCKS GROWTH
NOW Foods Maca
Total Curve Gel
Breast Success Cream

BODY MASS INDEX (BMI)

Supplements are a beneficial addition to a proper diet in reducing weight. Research shows that chromium picolinate and 5-HTP effectively promote weight loss in women. Herbal supplements may also be helpful for appetite control. Chromium deficiency is common in North America and may increase cravings for sweets. Chromium is known to regulate blood sugar levels and reduce cravings for sweets. 5-HTP increases serotonin levels in the brain. Serotonin deficiency is associated with the brain's perception of starvation and hunger.

Hoodia gordonii is an appetite suppressant. A Dutch anthropologist studying the primitive San Bushmen of the Kalahari Desert noticed that they ate the stem of the hoodia plant to suppress hunger during long hunting trips. The active ingredient in hoodia is the appetite-suppressing molecule P57. Scientists found that P57 acts on the brain in a manner similar to glucose. It tricks the brain into thinking you are full even when you have not eaten, reduces interest in food, and delays the time before hunger sets in. Women with diabetes should not use hoodia.

Garcinia cambogia contains a component called hydroxycitric acid (HCA) that suppresses the appetite and reduces the body's ability to form fatty tissue.

Guarana works in much the same way coffee does due to high levels of caffeine. Caffeine impairs the appetite. A study found that guarana improved memory, mood, and alertness. The lower dose of 75 milligrams produced more positive cognitive effects than the higher doses.

Ephedra sinica has thermogenic (fat burning) properties and is an excellent appetite suppressant. However, ephedra has some major safety concerns, including high blood pressure, tachycardia, CNS excitation, arrhythmia, heart attack, and stroke. It is not recommended unless under strict monitoring by a doctor.

WEIGHT-LOSS SUPPLEMENTS
Now Foods Chromium Picolinate
PES Alpha-T2
USP Labs OxyElite Pro
USP Labs Recreate
Primaforce Yohimbine HCI
BSN Atro-Phex
Now Foods Green Tea Extract
Natrol AcaiBerry Diet Acai & Green Tea Super Foods
Genesis Today Pure Green Coffee Bean
Hollywood Diet Hollywood 48-Hour Miracle Diet
Natrol Tonalin CLA
Michael's Naturopathic Ultimate Diet & Energy Tablets

APPETITE SUPRESSANTS
Now Foods 5-HTP
Source Naturals Garcinia 1000
Natural Balance Guarana Extra Strength
Source Naturals Hoodia Complex
Competitive Edge Labs Suppress-C
Athletic Xtreme Slim Xtreme

THERMOGENICS
Sports One Ma Huang
Lipodrene
PES Alphamine
BSN Hyper Shred Thermodynamic Metabolic Activator
Universal Nutrition Ripped Fast

MEAL REPLACEMENT
The Ultimate Life The Ultimate Meal
Garden of Life Raw Meal Beyond Organic Meal Replacement Formula
Garden of Life Raw Protein Beyond Organic Protein Formula
Vega Complete Whole Food Health Optimizer
Nature's Way Metabolic ReSet
Greens Plus Chia Omega 3 Energy Bar

WEIGHT-LOSS DEVICES

Gazelle Edge
LifeSpan Fitness VP-1000 Vibration Plate
The Flex Belt
The Flex Mini
Breathslim
Fit Bit Zip
Zaggora HotPants

Chapter 6: Breasts

When they [breasts] are huge, you become very self-conscious...I've learned something though, through my years of pondering and pontificating, and that is: men love them, and I love that.
- Drew Barrymore, American actress

Breast growth occurs most efficiently with the balanced presence of estrogen, progesterone, prolactin, human growth hormone (HGH), and growth factor (GF). After puberty, when the body ceases to produce a significant amount of these hormones, breast growth ends. By supplementing these hormones, breasts can grow even during adulthood. Hormone testing should be done to determine the most appropriate natural breast enlargement program to follow.

A breast enlargement program consisting of herbs, glandular therapy, or suction devices can be used to enlarge the breasts naturally. However, they may take two to four years of consistent effort to achieve desired results.

TOP BREAST ENHANCEMENT BRANDS
St Herb
www.stherb.com

Green Bush
www.greenbush.net

Nature's Way
www.naturesway.com

Now Foods
www.nowfoods.com

NATURAL BREAST ENLARGEMENT

Try each breast enlargement program for a minimum of one full year. When little improvement is seen after one year, move on to the next program. Choose only one program to follow, but don't mix and combine supplements from other programs because this will confuse the body and cause problems with hormonal balance.

Take phytoestrogens on an empty stomach or wait two to three hours after eating to take them. Bovine ovary is best taken with food. Spread out supplement doses throughout the day.

During any natural breast enlargement program, regular cleansing breaks are necessary for regulating hormonal levels. Follow each breast enlargement program for three months followed by a one month cleansing break. A cleansing break should consist of using only milk thistle, S-Adenosyl methionine (SAM), and 200 milligrams of diindolylmethane (DIM) once per day. Women that are on an estrogen program can also take the herb vitex as directed on the label.

Estrogen Metabolism Assessment is a test that evaluates how estrogen is being processed in the body and should be taken every four to five months. A Female Comprehensive Hormone Panel Blood Test should be taken every six to eight months to identify hormone imbalances that may result from a breast enlargement program.

Many women get permanent results, but some have needed to use a maintenance dosage of 100 milligrams of bovine ovary or 100 milligrams of each phytoestrogen per day after following a breast growth program for a few years.

Many women have enlarged breasts using a breast suction device. Like any tissue in the body, when the breasts are exercised and blood flow encouraged, they will enlarge. A suction device can be used instead of supplements, or along with supplements, to maximize breast growth. However, suction devices should not be used excessively or they could leave permanent indentations.

Massaging phytoestrogens into the breasts is an effective method for enlarging the breasts. Commercially prepared breast enlargement creams are available.

PHYTOESTROGEN
Premium Pueraria Mirifica
Biovea Pueraria Mirifica
St Herb Pueraria Mirifica
Green Bush Breast Enlargement Kit
Nature's Way Hops Flowers
Nature's Way Fennel Seed
Nature's Way Fenugreek Seed
Savesta Shatavari

GLANDULAR
Swanson Premium Raw Ovarian Glandular
Allergy Research Group Ovary Beef Natural Glandular

GALACTAGOGUE

Motherlove Goat's Rue
Nature's Wonderland Goat's Rue

PROGESTERONE
Nature's Herbs Mexican Wild Yam
Nature's Way Wild Yam

ANTIANDROGEN
Jarrow Formulas Saw Palmetto
Nature's Way Saw Palmetto Berries
Now Foods Saw Palmetto Berries
Eclectic Institute Saw Palmetto
Doctor's Best Best Saw Palmetto Standardized Extract
David's Tea Organic Spearmint

GROWTH SUPPORT
Symbiotics Colostrum Plus
21st Century Health Care Colostrum
GenF20Plus HGH Releaser
Source Naturals HGH Surge
Jarrow Formulas Whey Protein Ultrafiltered Powder
Source Naturals MSM Powder with Vitamin C
Doctor's Best Best MSM
Nature's Bounty Gelatin
Jarrow Formulas Certified Organic Flaxseed Oil
Natural Factors Omega Factors Flaxseed Oil
Now Foods Borage Oil
Nature's Way Alive! Whole Food Energizer Multi-Vitamin
Nature's Way Kelp

BREAST SUCTION DEVICES
Noogleberry
Bosom Beauty
Brava System

BREAST GROWTH CREAM
St Herb Nano Breast Cream
Biovea Pueraria Mirifica Breast Cream
Ainterol Pueraria Mirifica Breast Cream
Violetta's Garden Fenugreek Cream
Eclectic Institute Fenugreek
Indian Meadow Herbals Organic Wild Yam Root Cream
MoonMaid Botanicals ProMeno Wild Yam Cream
Now Foods Solutions Natural Progesterone Liposomal Skin Cream
Emerita Pro-Gest Cream

CLEANSING BREAK
Nature's Way DIM-plus Estrogen Metabolism Formula
Now Foods Indole-3-Carbinol
Jarrow Formulas Natural SAM-e 200
Now Foods Silymarin Milk Thistle Extract 2X

BREAST FIRMING PRODUCTS

Breasts need proper support during activity to maintain firmness. When breasts bounce during active sports, such as tennis or jogging, the Cooper's ligaments within the breasts can become stretched or even torn. A good sports bra can help prevent this.

Nutritional supplements may be helpful in slowing or preventing the progress of sagging breasts. However, supplements cannot reverse sagging breasts. Vitamin C and MSM are very important for collagen synthesis, which helps the Cooper's ligaments maintain the structural integrity of the breasts. Supplementing with collagen and essential fatty acids (EFAs) may also be helpful.

SPORTS BRA
Moving Comfort Fiona Bra
Enell High Impact Sports Bra
Glamorise Adjustable Motion Control Sports Bra
Danskin Now Sport Bra
Triumph Triaction Extreme Sports Bra
Nike Pro Victory Compression Sports Bra
Panache Maximum Control Ultimate Underwire Sports Bra
Champion Powerback Underwire Sports Bra
Freya Firm Control Underwire Sports Bra
Anita Extreme Control Sport Bra
Shock Absorber Ultimate Run Bra
Wacoal Sport Underwire Bra
Goddess Soft Cup Sports Bra

BREAST FIRMING CREAM
St Herb Nano Plus Breast Serum
Reviva Labs Elastin & Collagen Body Firming Lotion
Palmer's Cocoa Butter Formula Bust Cream
Avalon Organics CoQ10 Repair Ultimate Firming Body Lotion
Italiani Selex Busto-Lift Cream

BREAST FIRMING SUPPLEMENTS
Source Naturals MSM Powder with Vitamin C
Neocell Super Collagen+C Type 1 & 3
Jarrow Formulas Certified Organic Flaxseed Oil
Now Foods Borage Oil
Italiani Selex Busto-Lift Capsule

Chapter 7: Health

Health is the greatest gift
- Gautama Buddha, Spiritual teacher

The best place to find and purchase the selected health products in this chapter is on www.vitacost.com, www.iherb.com, www.amazon.com, www.longevitywarehouse.com, www.mynaturalmarket.com, or specific health brand website. To find various health devices and tools, go to www.toolsforwellness.com or www.trianglehealingproducts.com. *Osumex* (www.osumex.com) has easy to use health test kits.

Organic food can be purchased at local farmer's markets. Organic grocery delivery is another great option. Search the term "organic food delivery" on www.google.com. To find organic, grass-fed meat and dairy, go to www.eatwild.com and www.realmilk.com/where03.html.

While it is best to use natural health products, drugs can be helpful, especially during emergencies or during travel. Go to www.medify.com to find effective drugs and www.treato.com to view ratings.

TOP HEALTH SUPPLEMENT BRANDS
Primer Research Labs
www.shop.prlabs.com

Now Foods
www.nowfoods.com

Nature's Way
www.naturesway.com

Doctor's Best
www.drbvitamins.com

Eclectic Institute
www.eclecticherb.com

REMEDIES

Although conventional medicine is most effective for relief of severe pain, there are natural remedies available for the relief and prevention of mild to moderate pain.

Informed women take herb white willow bark instead of aspirin because it does not appear to be as irritating to the stomach lining and is more effective than aspirin because of other active compounds that are found in the whole herb but not the drug. Meadowsweet is an herb that is useful for joint and muscle pain relief. Magnesium, 5-HTP, feverfew, and butterbur are useful for headaches and migraines.

Peppermint is one of the world's oldest medicinal herbs and is scientifically proven to be effective for relieving headaches when applied topically to the temples and forehead.

CMO (cerasomal-cis-9-cetylmyristoleate) is a naturally derived substance that may be effective for all forms of arthritis, especially osteoarthritis and rheumatoid arthritis. CMO treats the cause of arthritis by reprogramming the immune system so that it no longer views its own tissues as foreign, and stops attacking them.

Yunnan Baiyao, taken internally, inhibits internal bleeding due to trauma, surgery or cerebral hemorrhage. It is useful for any type of open wound and any kind of surgery. It reduces recovery time for surgery by half because it mends injured blood vessels. It does not interfere with Western sedative drugs, so can be used the same day as surgery.

The use of antistress herbs will reduce the chances of developing a stress-related disease during periods of high stress or for those with a high-stress lifestyle. There are two types of herbs that are helpful for stress: Adaptogenic herbs improve energy; they support the organs and systems affected by stress, causing the body to become more resistant to stress. Calming herbs have a positive effect on the nervous system; they may reduce feelings of nervousness, anxiety, stress, and insomnia.

At times, energy levels may be low due to stress, excessive work, or lack of sleep, and quick energy boosts are required. Instead of consuming energy drinks, which are filled with sugar and artificial additives, get the specific energy-boosting nutrients from supplements. Caffeine, taurine, glucuronolactone, D-ribose, carnitine, guarana, ephedra, NADH, B vitamins, reduce tiredness.

When the immune system is compromised due to stress, the body no longer has full protection against illness. During high-stress periods, it is important to quickly boost immune strength. Research shows that certain herbs, extracts, and nutrients boost the immune system and are effective in preventing and treating colds and flu.

The Bible foretells a time when not having children will be considered a blessing. "For the days are coming when they will say, 'Fortunate indeed are the women who are childless, the wombs that have not borne a child and the breasts that have never nursed'" (NLT, Luke 23:29).

Finding an effective and safe method of birth control is important because it impacts a woman's health. Learn more about various methods of birth control at www.plannedparenthood.org/health-topics/birth-control-4211.htm.

Reversible Inhibition of Sperm Under Guidance (RISUG), also known as *Vasagel*, is a spermicidal polymer gel injected into the vas deferens. It blocks the tube and also kills any sperm that get past. It is one hundred percent effective at preventing pregnancy, completely reversible, and with virtually no serious side effects. It lasts about ten years.

Essure is a permanent, non-surgical way to block the fallopian tubes. For every 1,000 women who have *Essure*, fewer than 3 will become pregnant. If you might want to have children in the future, then the *Essure* procedure may not be right for.

The birth control implant, known as *Nexplanon*, is a thin, flexible plastic implant about the size of a cardboard matchstick. It is inserted under the skin of the upper arm. The progestin in the birth control implant works by keeping eggs from leaving the ovaries and making a woman's cervical mucus thicker. This keeps sperm from getting to the eggs. Less than 1 out of 100 women a year will become pregnant using the implant. It protects against pregnancy for up to three years.

An intrauterine device (IUD) is a small, "T-shaped" device inserted into the uterus to prevent pregnancy. It is considered safe, effective, and long lasting. Less than 1 out of 100 women will get pregnant each year using an IUD. Although the IUD is an effective method of birth control, it can come out of place and therefore should be checked regularly to be sure it is in place. The *ParaGard* IUD contains copper and is effective for 12 years. The *Mirena* IUD releases a small amount of progestin and is effective for five years. Both the *ParaGard* IUD and the *Mirena* IUDs work mainly by affecting the way sperm move so they can't join with an egg. The *ParaGard* IUD does not change a woman's hormone levels. The *Mirena* IUD may reduce period cramps and make periods lighter.

The emergency contraception pill (ECP), commonly called the morning-after pill, is a way to prevent pregnancy after unprotected sex. Levonorgestrel (*Plan B*) can be used up to 72 hours after having unprotected sex. Levonorgestrel works by giving high doses of the hormones estrogen and progesterone to prevent pregnancy. The other type, ulipristal acetate (*Ella*) can be taken up to 5 days after unprotected intercourse. *Ella* contains ulipristal, a non-hormonal drug that blocks the effects of key hormones necessary for conception. *Plan B* is sold without a prescription, while *Ella* is available only by prescription.

PAIN RELIEF REMEDIES
Now Foods White Willow Bark
Now Foods Feverfew
Now Foods Butterbur
Doctor's Best Magnesium High Absorption
Now Foods 5-HTP
Herb Pharm Meadowsweet
Now Foods Essential Oils 100% Pure Peppermint
CMO II
ActiveHerb Yunnan Baiyao

ANTISTRESS REMEDIES
Now Foods American Ginseng
Country Life Ginseng Supreme Complex

Nature's Way Schizandra Fruit
Now Foods Ashwagandha
Now Foods Rhodiola
Solaray Passion Flower
Eclectic Institute Kava Whole Lateral Root
Now Foods Valerian Root
Eclectic Institute Skullcap Organic
Eclectic Institute Motherwort Organic

IMMUNE BOOSTING REMEDIES
Source Naturals Wellness Formula Herbal Defense Complex
Garden of Life Primal Defense HSO Probiotic Formula
Madre Labs Immune Punch
NutriBiotic DefensePlus Maximum Strength
Now Foods Total Well-Being
Now Foods Immune Renew
Nature's Way Echinacea Goldenseal
Now Foods Astragalus
Now Foods Cat's Claw Extract
Nature's Way Suma, Root
Now Foods Oregano Oil
Mannatech Ambrotose
Paradise Herbs Ultimate Andrographis
Nature's Way Zinc Lozenges
Zand Elderberry Zinc Herbalozenge
Herb Pharm Mistletoe
Boiron Oscillococcinum
Boiron Influenzinum
Now Foods Olive Leaf Extract
NutriBiotic DefensePlus Grapefruit Seed Extract
Allimax 100% Allicin Powder Capsules
Wakunaga Kyolic Aged Garlic Extract Immune Formula
Fungi Perfecti Host Defense MyCommunity
Nutricology ImmoPlex Glandular
Nutricology Thymus
Macrolife Naturals Macro Greens Nutrient Rich Super-Food
Himalaya Herbal Healthcare Organic Chyavanprash
Source Naturals DMG
Nature's Way Alive! Vitamin C 100% Whole Food Complex
Source Naturals N-Acetyl Cysteine
Garden of Life Vitamin Code Raw B-Complex
Source Naturals Wellness Colloidal Silver Throat Spray
Symbiotics Colostrum Plus
Quantum Nutrition Labs Quantum-RX Nucleotides

ENERGY-BOOSTING REMEDIES
Living Essentials 5 Hour Energy
Now Foods Energy
Purecaf Liquid Caffeine
5150 Juice Liquid Caffeine
Prolab Nutrition Caffeine

Chi-Tea Organic Green Tea Caffeine
Doctor's Best Chewable D-Ribose
Now Foods Taurine
Serious Nutrition Solution Glucuronolactone
Doctor's Best Best L-Carnitine Fumarate
Natural Balance Guarana Extra Strength
Hi-tech Pharmaceuticals Black Widow
Natrol NADH Maximum Strength
New Chapter Organics Coenzyme B Food Complex
MegaFood DailyFoods Balanced B Complex

BIRTH CONTROL METHODS
Vasagel
Essure
Nexplanon
ParaGard IUD / *Mirena* IUD
Plan B / *Ella*

NUTRITIONAL SUPPLEMENTS

Providing adequate nourishment to the body will prevent diseases. Studies show that inadequate intake of several vitamins is associated with chronic disease. Taking a whole food supplement daily is highly recommended. Many naturopaths and health care professionals also recommend taking extra vitamin D and vitamin C supplements.

Whole food supplements are made from concentrated whole foods. A whole food supplement is better absorbed and assimilated by the body than synthetic supplements.

A great way to get sufficient minerals is through juicing organic vegetables. Invest in a high quality masticating juicer, and then juice a variety of different vegetables every day. A masticating juicer eliminates the fiber from vegetables and leaves only the concentrated nutrients. You can juice apple, pear, pomegranate, kiwi, carrot, broccoli, beet, kale, Swiss chard, collard greens, spinach, celery, cucumber, cabbage, parsley, arugula, dandelion greens, watercress, wheatgrass, and ginger. Besides juicing, take ionic minerals. Ionic minerals are 10,000 times smaller than colloidal minerals.

Spirulina and chlorella are highly nutritious and a rich source of minerals. Spirulina is about 51–71 percent protein, depending on its source. It is a complete protein containing all essential amino acids. There are many health benefits of spirulina for immunomodulation, anticancer, antiviral, and cholesterol-reduction effects.

Essential amino acids are not produced by the body and need to be taken in through diet or supplements. Vegans are especially at risk of developing an amino acid deficiency. The nine essential amino acids are: histidine, isoleucine, leucine, lysine, methionine, phenylalanine, threonine, tryptophan, and valine. Free-form amino acid supplements are the best. Free-form amino acids don't require digestion. The term "free-form" means the amino acids move quickly through the stomach

-

and into the small intestine, where they're rapidly absorbed into the bloodstream.

Essential fatty acids (EFAs) are nutrients that humans need to obtain from food or supplements because the body cannot synthesize them and requires them for good health. Supplementing omega-3 is very important since many holistic health experts agree that many illnesses are associated with a deficiency of omega-3 fatty acids. Omega-3 is best obtained through wild salmon oil, cod-liver oil, or krill oil. Flaxseed oil can be included in the diet but is not the best source for essential fatty acids (EFAs).

One of the main causes of disease is oxygen deficiency. Active oxygen (O1) supplements are superior to any drug, herb, or latest health technology in preventing and treating illness.

An overwhelming amount of research has firmly established that the consumption of berry fruits prevents disease and improves health. Exotic superberries such mangosteen, mulberry, noni, goji, and acai have many health benefits and build disease resistance.

A healthy liver is vital to good health. There are numerous diseases and conditions that are associated with a weakened, damaged, or diseased liver. All encounter some threat of damage or disease to the liver due to environmental pollution, poor eating habits, alcohol, and pharmaceutical drugs use. Women with liver conditions or a poorly functioning liver can support the liver on a daily basis.

Herbal elixirs such as Chinese foxglove root, cistanche, shilajit, chyawanprash are designed to prevent disease and aging can be consumed daily. Indian and Chinese civilizations are experts in their production and use. A traditional Chinese medicine (TCM) doctor or Indian herbalist can devise the perfect formulation specifically designed for each individual woman.

Precaution is essential during travel since travel exposes the body to infections unknown to the immune system. Every woman should have a travel health kit that consists of echinacea, charcoal tablets, probiotics, antibiotics, antivirotics, goldenseal, garlic capsules, colloidal silver, and food grade hydrogen peroxide.

Go to a travel clinic and visit www.cdc.gov/travel/ or www.tripprep.com before your trip to determine which immunizations are appropriate for your country of destination. Travelers may receive immunizations for hepatitis, meningococcal infection, typhoid fever, or yellow fever, as well as any vaccinations in the regular immunization schedule that the person may have missed or may need to renew, such as those for diphtheria and tetanus.

Be sure to stock up on appropriate antivirotics and antibiotics for preventing or treating common infectious diseases acquired during travel. Infectious diseases can be caused by bacterial, viral, fungal, or parasitic microorganisms and contributes to millions of deaths each year.

Sumycin, known as tetracycline, is a broad-spectrum antibiotic, active against a wide variety of bacteria. It is effective against E. coli and salmonella infections as well as cholera and typhus.

Rocephin is a broad-spectrum antibiotic, used to prevent and treat many kinds of bacterial infections, including severe or life-threatening forms such as meningitis.

Cipro is used to treat or prevent certain infections caused by bacteria. *Cipro* is also used to treat or prevent anthrax in people who may have been exposed to anthrax germs in the air. It can also be used to treat some forms of infectious diarrhea, and typhoid fever.

Doryx, known as doxycycline, is used to treat bacterial infections, including pneumonia and other respiratory tract infections; Lyme disease; and anthrax. It is also used to prevent and treat malaria.

Lariam and *Malarone* are used to treat malaria (a serious infection that is spread by mosquitoes in certain parts of the world and can cause death) and to prevent malaria in travelers who visit areas where malaria is common. Some people prefer taking *Lariam* and others prefer *Malarone*.

Primaquine is used to treat malaria in an infected person and to prevent the disease from coming back in people that are infected with malaria. *Primaquine* is used after other medications (*Malarone* or *Aralen*) have killed the malaria parasites living inside red blood cells. *Primaquine* kills the malaria parasites living in other body tissues. *Primaquine* combined with *Malarone* or *Aralen* are needed for a complete cure.

Dukoral is an oral vaccine that provides protection against intestinal infection caused by enterotoxigenic E. coli (ETEC) and cholera. Almost every developing country faces cholera outbreaks and the threat of a cholera epidemic, especially South American and African countries, India, Dominican Republic, and Haiti. *Dukoral* is available from a pharmacy or travel clinic.

Two *Pepto-Bismol* tablets taken four times per day can decrease the incidence of intestinal infection by about 60%. One or two *Imodium* tablets every four hours as needed can reduce the symptoms of intestinal infection.

Antibiotics don't work against viruses. Antivirotics, commonly known as antiviral drugs, are effective again viral infections. They work by inhibiting the development of the virus. Like antibiotics, specific antivirotics are used for specific viruses. In the future, broad-spectrum antiviral drugs that kills a variety of viruses will become available. DRACO is an experimental antiviral drugs under development at the Massachusetts Institute of Technology. DRACO is reported to have broad-spectrum efficacy against many infectious viruses. Until broad-spectrum antiviral drugs become available, stock up on antiviral drugs that treat common viruses that travelers may encounter.

Moroxydine broad-spectrum antiviral drugs used for the prevention and treatment of influenza. It is effective against a number of DNA and RNA viruses.

Rebetol, known as ribavirin, is an anti-viral drug that is effective in treating many viral infections. It is used to treat severe RSV infection, hepatitis C infection (used with peginterferon alfa-2b or peginterferon alfa-2a), SARS, and other viral infections.

Tamiflu is used for the prevention and treatment of Influenza A and Influenza B including swine flu H1N1 virus. It works to slow the spread of influenza (flu) virus between cells in the body.

Relenza is an inhaled medication used for treating and preventing influenza, including H1N1. *Relenza* suppresses and decreases the spread of influenza A and B viruses. It helps shorten the symptoms and duration of influenza infection.

Alinia, known as nitazoxanide, is an antiparasitic medicine, particularly effective against giardiasis and cryptosporidiosis. It can treat hepatitis C, in combination with peginterferon alfa-2a and ribavirin.

Ideally, before seeking treatment for infection, you should identify the type of bacterial or viral infection in your body. Hospitals typically have a Division of Microbiology that provides laboratory services to patients. Real-time PCR (qPCR) will accurately diagnosis infectious diseases. Once you have identified the type of infection, you can select appropriate treatment.

In the near future, researchers will create a portable DNA detection device that will determine which type of virus or bacteria is in your body and also reveal how much is present. In their most recent research, Dr. Yi Lu, Ph.D., and Yu Xiang converted a glucose meter (used by diabetes patients to check blood sugar) into a device that could monitor DNA. This device could become a cheap and easy way to perform tests for viruses and bacteria at home or during travel. For now, larger systems used by researchers are available such as Eco Real-Time PCR System available at www.ecoqpcr.com.

Following a radiological or nuclear event, radioactive iodine may be released into the air and then be breathed into the lungs. Radioactive iodine may also contaminate the local food supply and get into the body through food or through drink. The thyroid gland quickly absorbs radioactive iodine and can injure the gland. Potassium iodide works to block radioactive iodine from being taken into the thyroid gland and can help protect this gland from injury. Adults should take 130 mg to protect themselves. One capsule of *Club Natural* Potassium Iodide has 130 mg.

MASTICATING JUICER
Norwalk Juicer 280
Champion Juicer G5-PG710
*Omega J*8006 Juicer
Green Star GSE-5000 Elite
Super Angel 5500
Green Power KPE-1304
Breville 800JEXL Juice Fountain Elite
Kuvings NS-940

WHOLE FOOD SUPPLEMENTS
Phyto Vita Regulat
Nature's Way Alive! Whole Food Energizer Multi-Vitamin
Garden of Life Vitamin Code Women
MegaFood Women's One Daily
Nutricology ProGreens with Advanced Probiotic Formula
Quantum Nutrition Labs Daily Multi
Lumina Health Cell Food Oxygen Supplement

VITAMIN D
MegaFood Vitamin D3
Now Foods Vitamin D-3

Healthy Origins Vitamin D3
Nature's Answer Vitamin D-3 Drops
Doctor's Best Best Vitamin D3
Carlson Labs Vitamin D3

VITAMIN C
LivOn Laboratories Lypo-Spheric Vitamin C
Nature's Way Alive! Vitamin C
New Chapter Organics Activated C Food Complex
Madre Labs Madre-C Vitamin C
Pure Essence Whole C Whole Food Vitamin C
MegaFood Ultra C-400
Garden of Life Living Vitamin C
The Synergy Company Pure Radiance C

IONIC FULL-SPECTRUM MINERALS
Mr. Oxygen's OxyMins
Optimally Organic Fulvic Ionic Minerals
Trace Minerals Research ConcenTrace

SPIRULINA / CHLORELLA
Ergogenics Nutrition Organic Whole Greens
Garden of Life Perfect Food Super Green Formula
Now Foods Certified Organic Spirulina
Now Foods Certified Organic Chlorella

FREE-FORM AMINO ACIDS
NutraBio AminoPro Free-Form Amino Acid Complex
ProHealth Amino Acid Complex

ESSENTIAL FATTY ACIDS
Natural Factors Omega Factors Wild Alaskan Salmon Oil
New Chapter Wholemega Extra-Virgin Wild Alaskan Salmon
Solgar Full Spectrum Omega Wild Alaskan
Now Foods Cod Liver Oil Double Strength
Now Foods Neptune Krill Oil

ACTIVE OXYGEN
Mr. Oxygen's OxyLift
Dr. Wong's Essentials Stabilized Oxygen

SUPERBERRIES
Madre Labs Eureka! Berries
Life Time Noni Mangosteen Goji & Acai Blend
Natural Factors WellBetX Mulberry Extract

LIVER SUPPLEMENTS
Now Foods Silymarin Milk Thistle Extract 2X
Natural Factors Milk Thistle Extract
Nature's Way Thisilyn Liver Support Formula
Nature's Way Milk Thistle

Enzymatic Therapy Liv-A-Tox
Himalaya Herbal Healthcare Liver Care
Quantum Nutrition Labs Liver-PG
ActiveHerb Xiao Yao Wan
Chinese Natural Herbs Lung Dan Xie Gan Wan
Chinese Natural Herbs Lidan Tablets
Nature's Secret Milk Thistle Liver Cleanse
Cheung's Trading Mormodia & Oldenlandia Diffusa Tea
RXhomeo Nux Vomica
Pekana apo-hepat
Pekana Toxex

HERBAL ELIXIRS
TerraVita Chinese Foxglove
ActiveHerb Cistanche
Dragon Herbs High Mountain Shilajit
Himalaya Herbal Healthcare Organic Chyavanprash

TRAVEL SUPPLEMENTS
Eclectic Institute Echinacea Goldenseal Combination
Nature's Way Charcoal Activated
Now Foods Gr8-Dophilus
Wakunaga Kyolic Aged Garlic Extract Immune
Silver Mountain Minerals Colloidal Silver Ultra 240 ppm
OxyLife Stabilized Oxygen With Colloidal Silver

TRAVEL ANTIBIOTICS
Sumycin
Rocephin
Cipro
Lariam / Malarone
Doryx
Primaquine

TRAVEL ANTIVIROTICS
Moroxydine
Rebetol
Tamiflu
Relenza
Alinia

PURE WATER
2 Pure H2O Water System
Radiant Life 14-Stage Biocompatible Water Purification System
Joyfay Quartz Pure Water Distiller Auto-Threefold Triple Distillation
HuaShen Treasure Cup of Life
Oxy Water

HEALTHY HOME PRODUCTS

Every woman that cares about her health will get an EMF radiation-protection cell phone chip on her phone. A radiation-protection cell chip will neutralize harmful effects of EMR. Women can also wear a personal EMF protection shield in the form of a necklace or bracelet. All commonly used electronic devices such as laptops and tablet PCs should also have a protection chip applied onto it. Select a radiation-protection cell chip that is backed by research and testing.

The most important way the body regenerates is through rest and relaxation, which tends to be done in the home. Creating a healthy home environment will contribute to disease resistance.

EMF PROTECTION
EP2 Stress Pendant
eDot Cell Phone EMR Blocker
EMF-BioShield
Q-Link Pendant
Eradicator Technologies Lotus Shield
GIAlife Pendant
Cell Phone *Bioprotector*
Home and Office *Bioprotector*
EarthCalm Quantum Cell
EarthCalm Home Protection
HuaShen Card for Cellphone
HuaShen Energy Disc Pendant

ORGANIC MATTRESS
NaturaOrganics EcoSancturary Firm Mattress
Savvy Rest Serenity Mattress
Bella Sera Nove 3 Organic Mattress
Eco Brilliance Mattress
Life Kind The Traditional Mattress
Green Sleep Dolcezza Mattress

MAGNETIC MATTRESS PADS
Magna-Pak Magnetic Mattress Pad
Therion Magnetic Mattress Pad
Tools For Wellness Magnetic Mattress Pad

HEPA AIR PURIFIER
IQAIR
BLUEAIR
Austin Air
Alen Air Purifier

NON-TOXIC PAINT
Unearthed Paints
Silacote Paint
Bioshield Paint
Anna Sova Wall Paint
Auro Usa Paint
Real Milk Paint

Earthborn Eco Paint
Yolo Colorhouse
Green Planet Paints
Ecos Organic Paint
AFM Safecoat
Freshaire Choice
Olympic's Premium Paint

MAGNETIC RESONANCE STIMULATION
MediConsult iMRS Complete
QRS Quantron
Bemer 3000

Chapter 8: Style

Style is knowing who you are; what you want to say.
- Gore Vidal, American novelist

Nearly all the clothing designers selected in this chapter offer clothing staples constructed with high-quality natural fabrics such as wool, silk, or cotton in wearable, flattering styles. However, it is still important to check to see what fabrics were used to create each individual piece, because sometimes designers sneak in cheap, synthetic fabrics.

You can also find some designers items on www.polyvore.com or www.shopstyle.com where fabric content is usually listed. For disposable, fashionable clothing that only lasts a season or two, select items from *H&M* (www.hm.com), *Topshop* (www.topshop.com), *Warehouse* (www.warehouse.co.uk), or *Oasis* (www.oasis-stores.com).

TOP STYLE DESIGNERS
Jil Sander
www.jilsander.com

Hobbs
www.hobbs.co.uk

Akris
www.akris.ch

Valentino Garavani
www.valentino.com

Chinti and Parker
www.chintiandparker.com

CLOTHING

Sleeping in how the body regenerates. Therefore, it is especially important to wear sleepwear that is constructed with natural and breathable fabrics such as silk and organic cotton. Natural fabrics allow the skin to breathe which in turn promotes rejuvenation.

Visible bra lines and visible panty lines look very unstylish. *MySkins* Lingerie created seamless, invisible panties in skin-tone-matching colors that lay flat against the body. They remain undetectable underneath clothing. Strapless bras tend to slip down. Instead of wearing a strapless bra, wear a seamless, strapless bustier or overbust corset. Be sure to decide if you need a bustier or a corset as their function is different. A corset reduces the waist size, typically by two to four inches. An overbust bustier lifts up the breasts to create cleavage.

All the designers selected offer most clothing pieces constructed with natural fabrics and wearable styles. Selected clothing staples from these designers in classic colors so they never go out of style. Classic colors include white, beige, black, very dark gray, very dark blue, and red.

SLEEPWEAR
Agent Provocateur
Bodas
Jenny Packham
Beautiful Bottoms
Samantha Chang
Carine Gilson
Dana Pisarra
Mimi Holliday
La Fee Verte
Jean Yu
Skin
Gaiam
Faeries Dance

UNDERGARMENTS
Bazsarózsa
Beautiful Bottoms
Sonata Lingerie
Samantha Chang
Mimi Holliday
La Fee Verte
Faeries Dance
Couture Cottons
Pact
MySkins Lingerie
Lace Embrace
Sparklewren

SOCKS
Cottonique
Ecoland

Pact
Bleu Foret
Dore Dore

TOPS
Joseph
Chinti and Parker
Stewart + Brown
bgreen apparel
Indigenous Designs
Alice + Olivia
3.1 Phillip Lim
Moschino
Marc Jacobs
Ralph Lauren
Steffen Schraut
Closed
Enza Costa
Rag & Bone

SHORTS
Marc Jacobs
Ralph Lauren
Blumarine
Citizens of Humanity
Rag & Bone
Diane von Furstenberg
Burberry

PANTS
Closed
Chinti and Parker
Allison Wonderland
Hobbs
Diane von Furstenberg
The Row
Joseph
Rachel Zoe
Isabel Marant
Haider Ackermann
Brunello Cucinelli
Elie Saab
Emilio Pucci

JEANS
Nudie Jeans
Monkee Genes
Chloé
Zara
Citizens of Humanity
Rag & Bone

Current/Elliott
Hudson
Ralph Lauren
Seven
J Brand Jeans
Burberry

SKIRTS
Chinti and Parker
Allison Wonderland
David Koma
Jil Sander
Hobbs
Joseph
Jason Wu
Elie Saab
Ralph Lauren
Valentino Garavani
Prabal Gurung
Roksanda Ilincic
Reiss
Marc Jacobs
Ralph Lauren
MaxMara
Blumarine
Joseph
Alexander McQueen
Oscar de la Renta
Prabal Gurung
Diane von Furstenberg
The Row
Akris
Steffen Schraut
Haider Ackermann
Giambattista Valli
Whistles
Maxmara
Emilio Pucci

DRESSES
Elie Saab
Orla Kiely
Chinti and Parker
Stewart + Brown
Allison Wonderland
Issa
Libélula
Jenny Packham
Joseph
Jason Wu
Alexander McQueen

Erdem
Pamella Roland
Jean Fares Couture
Pamela Dennis
John Galliano
Zuhair Murad
Matthew Williamson
Erdem
Roksanda Ilincic
Sherri Hill
Tony Bowls
Terani Couture
Jovani
La Femme
Alyce Designs
Ralph Lauren
Blumarine
The Blonds
Zimmermann
Roland Mouret
Oscar de la Renta
Prabal Gurung
Diane von Furstenberg
Emilia Wickstead
Giambattista Valli
Temperley
Alberta Ferretti
Matthew Williamson
Leonard
Pendleton

SWEATERS
Chinti and Parker
Stewart + Brown
Erdaine Knitwear
360 Sweater
Jil Sander
Joseph
Ralph Lauren
Closed
Joseph
Crumpet
Zenggi
Enza Costa
Valentino Garavani
Stefanel
Minnie Rose
Moschino
Isabel Marant
Maxmara
Temperley

Tara Jarmon
Matthew Williamson
Malo
Pendleton

COATS / JACKETS
Joseph
Libélula
Katherine Hooker
Burberry
Blumarine
Yves Saint Laurent
Roland Mouret
L.K. Bennett
L'Wren Scott
Emilio Pucci

WEDDING

For wedding dresses, many women may prefer to purchase a pre-owned wedding dress. You're reducing your environmental impact by re-using a wedding dress. It's also cost-effective since it's only been worn once and looks like a brand new dress for half the price. The best place to find pre-owned wedding dress online is www.preownedweddingdresses.com or www.oncewed.com/used-wedding-dresses. Some women may prefer to order custom made wedding dresses from chosen bridal dress designer listed.

WEDDING DRESSES
Yumi Katsura Couture
Jenny Packham
Alexander McQueen
Vera Wang
John Galliano
Simone Carvalli
Justin Alexander
Hayley Paige
Maggie Sottero
Mori Lee
Eddy K
Jim Hjelm
Paula Varsalona
Alex Perry
Alma Novia

SHOES

The shoe designers selected construct some or most of their shoes with leather or suede upper, lining, insole, and outsole. For women who are conscious of animal rights and refuse to wear anything animal, then vegan shoes are available from www.mooshoes.com or the designer *Olsen Haus* (www.olsenhaus.com).

DESIGNER SHOES
Alexander Mcqueen
Jimmy Choo
Stuart Weitzman
Christian Louboutin
Manolo Blahnik
Brian Atwood
Diane Von Furstenberg
Kate Spade
Charlotte Olympia
Sergio Rossi
Nicholas Kirkwood
Giuseppe Zanotti
Yves Saint Laurent
Alice + Olivia
Aruna Seth
Bottega Veneta
Burberry
Cole Haan
Vera Wang
Tory Burch
Badgley Mischka
L.K. Bennett

ACCESSORIES

All the purses, gloves, scarves, and hats selected are designed with natural, quality fabrics such as silk, cotton, and animal skin. The jewelry designers are well respected and offer high-quality jewelry. The sunglasses selected are well constructed and use high-quality materials in their design.

The nail polishes are natural and non-toxic and some are even beneficial to the nails such as *Dr.'s Remedy* Enriched Nail Polish, which works to strengthen and nourish the nails. *Dr.'s Remedy* Enriched Nail Polish contains vitamins C and E as well as garlic bulb extract and tea tree oil.

Water-based nail polish such as *Suncoat* Nail Polish, *Honeybee Gardens* Watercolors, *Acquarella* Nail Polish don't contain any dangerous chemical solvents. Water-based nail polish is non-toxic, don't smell, and don't damage the nails.

Zoya Nail Polish is free of toluene, formaldehyde and dibutylphalate (DBP). It still may smell though. There are many beautiful colors to choose from.

OPI Nail Polish is free of DBP, toluene and formaldehyde. It goes on smoothly and lasts fairly long. It has many colors to choose from. The majority of women have been very happy with this nail polish brand.

Nailene Sensationail Color Gel Polish lasts up to two weeks, don't chip, and stays shiny. It can last up to three month on the toes. It goes on smooth and completely dries within two minutes. It may be difficult to remove.

CND Shellac is gel polish best applied by a top rated manicurist. It is painted onto the nail and dries hard like a fake nail. It lasts for two weeks and doesn't chip.

Innocent Oils Pinkie Drops Cuticle & Nail Oil nourishes, softens cuticles, nails and skin. It is best used every week. Use it two times per day to repair dry cuticles and nails.

Sephora Collection Express Nail Polish Remover does not contain parabens, sulfates, phthalates, GMOs and triclosan. It removes nail polish very effectively and quickly. It has no strong smell.

PURSES
Maison du Posh
Emilio Pucci
Yves Saint Laurent
Alexander McQueen
Chanel
Brahmin
Givenchy
Zagliani
Salvatore Ferragamo
Anya Hindmarch
3.1 Phillip Lim
Mulberry
Fendi
Karen Millen
Valentino Garavani
Diane Von Furstenberg
Paul Smith
Zara
Dolce & Gabbana
Nancy Gonzalez
Vivienne Westwood
Marni
Chloe
Gucci
Tod's
Marc Jacobs
Aspinal of London

OPERA GLOVES
Yves Saint Laurent
Diane Von Furstenberg
Portolano
Aspinal of London
Lanvin

SCARVES

Alexander Mcqueen
Aspinal of London
Valentino Garavani
Yves Saint Laurent
Emilio Pucci
Brooks Brothers
Gucci
Mermi
Erdem
Jimmy Choo
Shawlux
Bonana van Mil
Burberry
Givenchy
Marc Jacobs
Diane Von Furstenberg
Peter Pilotto
Matthew Williamson
Leonard
Beck Sonder Gaard
Janie Besner
Bajra
Yuh Okano

HATS
Rag & Bone
Marzi Firenze
Aspinal of London
Jane Corbett
Rachel Trevor-Morgan
Whiteley
Ann-Marie Faulkner Millinery
Anne-Sophie Coulot
Bundle MacLaren Millinery
Lock & Co Hatters Sylvia Fletcher
Jane Taylor Millinery
Philip Treacy
Laurence Leleux
Kokin Hat
Betmar Plaza Suite
Patricia Underwood
Yvette Jelfs
Helen Kaminski

SUNGLASSES
Judith Leiber
Chopard
Feri
Oakley
Ray-Ban
Luxuriator

Chrome Hearts

JEWELERY
Martin Katz
Harry Winston
Garrard & Co
Chopard
De Beers
Graff Diamonds
Neil Lane
Heavenly Necklaces

NAILS
Dr.'s Remedy Enriched Nail Polish
Suncoat Nail Polish
Honeybee Gardens Watercolors
Acquarella Nail Polish
Zoya Nail Polish
OPI Nail Polish
Sally Hansen Salon Effects Nail Polish Strips
CND Shellac
Innocent Oils Pinkie Drops Cuticle & Nail Oil
Sephora Collection Express Nail Polish Remover

SCENT

The best-reviewed perfumes were selected from www.makeupalley.com regardless of their ingredients. Unlike most products selected in this book, the perfumes are not completely natural and healthy, but if worn once in a while, they do little harm. If you prefer wearing an organic and natural scent you can wear essential oils, or purchase perfume from an organic perfumer.

PERFUMES
Chanel Coco Mademoiselle
Burberry Classic EDP
Stella McCartney Stella
Jovan Woman

ORGANIC PERFUMES
Aftelier Perfumes
Tsi~La Natural Perfumery & Organics
Skindecent Scents
Ajne Organic Scents
Honoré des Prés
Intelligent Nutrients Aromatics

ESSENTIAL OIL SCENTS
Aura Cacia
Essential Aura

Young Living
Eden Botanicals
Now Foods Essential Oils
Primavera Essential Oils

Chapter 9: Personality

When people see your personality come out, they feel so good, like
they actually know who you are.
- Usain Bolt, Jamaican athlete

"The 'self-image' is the key to human personality and human behavior.
Change the self-image and you change the personality and the
behavior," said American scientist Maxwell Maltz. Therefore, start by
changing your self-image with affirmations. You can resort to personality
supplements when affirmations are not enough to change the personality
and the behavior.

Before determining supplements to take for the personality, first
determine the root cause of personality problems. Start by taking a
Rorschach test, which is a psychological test in which subjects'
perceptions of inkblots are recorded and then analyzed to examine a
person's personality characteristics and emotional functioning. Then take
further tests such as a medical intuitive scan, quantum biofeedback, or
aura imagery to help determine the cause of negative personality traits.
Once a cause is found, an appropriate supplement can be selected.

TOP PERSONALITY SUPPLEMENT BRANDS
FES Quintessentials
www.fesflowers.com

Bach Essence
www.bachflower.com

Rxhomeo
www.rxhomeo.com

Vaxa International
www.vaxa.com

BEHAVIOR

Once you have determined the behavior to change, use kinesiology, also known as muscle testing, to determine which supplements will be effective in changing the behavior. Test all the supplements listed in a specific category to determine which one will work best.

ANTI-ANGER
Now Foods L-Tyrosine
FES Quintessentials Snapdragon
Hyland's Nux Vomica
Dhealth Store Anti-Anger Elixir

ANTIDEPRESSANTS
Now Foods 5-HTP
Doctor's Best SAM-e 400 Double-Strength
Doctor's Best Best Lithium Orotate
Now Foods Borage Oil
Now Foods Valerian Root
Rxhomeo Depression Relief Combo

ANTI-ANXIETY
Michael's Naturopathic Anxiety Relief / Stress
Jarrow Formulas StressTame
Now Foods GABA
Natural Vitality Natural Calm Plus Calcium
Eclectic Institute Skullcap
Now Foods Passion Flower Extract
Nature's Way Hops Flowers
Herb Pharm California Poppy
Rxhomeo Lycopodium
Rxhomeo Ignatia

CALMING
Bach Essence Rescue Remedy
Source Naturals Theanine Serene with Relora
Kira St. John's Wort
Vaxa International Nite-Rest
Natural Care SleepFix
NatraBio Insomnia Relief
Hyland's Calms Fortè
Nature's Way Melissa

COMMUNICATION

Kava kava extract is a sedative that is effective for reducing social anxiety and works in a similar way as alcohol to relax an individual during social interactions.

Propranolol is a sympatholytic non-selective beta blocker. Taken about an hour before any public presentation or interview, it reduces anxiety and panic as well as other symptoms associated with fear of public speaking. Many have commented that it is very effective. It does not have to take it everyday, only before speaking engagements. Users take between 10-40mg prior to a speech. Propranolol is available in generic form as propranolol hydrochloride, as well as under the brand names Inderal, Inderal LA, Avlocardyl, Deralin, Dociton, Inderalici, InnoPran XL, Sumial, Anaprilinum, and Bedranol SR.

Flower essences are subtle energy formulas that work to help the body, mind and spirit come into balance. They can be effectively used for those with public speaking difficulties. You can select suitable remedies on www.lichenwood.com/flower%20essences.html for negative emotions. Each flower essence can be taken individually or combined to be even more effective.

Cosmos flower essence is for those with rapid and inarticulate speech as well as difficulty communicating their ideas and beliefs to others. Cosmos aids the mind in organizing information so that it can be easily retrieved and expressed with coherence and clarity. It improves heartfelt communication, helping the personality shine forth.

Mimulus flower essence is for those with fear of public speaking, shuttering, nervousness, and shyness. It helps build courage and confidence. It promotes calmness and fluency of speech. Rock Rose might be preferred where the fear of public speaking causes terror.

Garlic flower essence is for those with fears, insecurities and lack of vital energy. It enables one to feel strong, stable, safe and secure. This essence protects the auric field.

Trumpet Vine helps those with an inability to speak clearly and lack of vitality in expression. It reduces stuttering. It allows those who are shy or intimidated to speak assertively and with a sense of self-empowerment. It promotes articulate and vibrant self-expression.

SPEAKING SKILLS
Now Foods Kava Kava Extract
Inderal (Propranolol)
FES Quintessentials Cosmos
Bach Essence Mimulus
FES Quintessentials Garlic
FES Quintessentials Trumpet Vine

INTELLIGENCE

Nootropics, also referred to as smart drugs or memory enhancers, are substances that improve intelligence, memory, attention, and concentration.

Acetylcholine is a neurotransmitter that is important for memory and learning. Acetylcholine deficiency can result in learning difficulties, memory problems, poor attention problems, and difficulty concentrating. Specific supplements such as Alpha-GPC and phosphatidylcholine can increase acetylcholine. Huperzine A helps preserve acetylcholine in the brain. Therefore, Alpha-GPC or phosphatidylcholine taken with Huperzine A may improve mental functioning.

Onnit Alpha Brain is an effective nootropics. It contains Alpha GPC, Huperzine A, Vinpocetine, AC-11, phosphatidylserine, bacopa, pterostilbene, l-tyrosine, l-theanine, oat straw, and vitamin B6.

Nature's Purest Brain Factors is a formula containing some of the most important cognitive enhancers. It contains acetyl l-carnitine, DMAE, Huperzine A, Alpha GPC, Vinpocetine, phosphatidylserine, ginkgo biloba leaf extract, and gotu kola herb extract.

Himalaya Herbal Healthcare MindCare helps improve memory, attention, and reduces mental fatigue. It contains a herbal blend of bacopa, gotu kola, dwarf morning glory, ashwagandha, jatamansi, Indian valerian, vidanga, almond, Indian tinospora, chebulic myrobalan, amla, oroxylum, celastrus, curculigo, velvet bean, cardamom, arjuna, fennel, finger-leaf morning glory, ginger, belleric myrobalan, nutmeg, and clove.

AOR Ortho Mind contains ingredients that help prevent memory impairment and improve mental focus. It contains vitamin B6, R-lipoic acid, bacopa monniera extract, ginkgo biloba extract, panax ginseng extract, citicoline cognizin, acetyl-l-carnitine HCl, and l-arginine-l-pyroglutamic acid.

The *Transparent Corp* Neuro-Programmer 3 is a software application that combines brainwave entrainment and applied psychology in one program to help enhance mental abilities. It is available from www.transparentcorp.com.

The *Brain Evolution System* uses brainwave entrainment to boost mental capacity and improve memory. It is available from www.brainev.com.

BRAIN ENHANCING SUPPLEMENTS
Onnit Alpha Brain
Nature's Purest Brain Factors
Himalaya Herbal Healthcare MindCare
AOR Ortho Mind

BRAIN ENHANCING DEVICES
Transparent Corp Neuro-Programmer 3
Brain Evolution System

Chapter 10: Character

Be more concerned with your character than your reputation, because your character is what you really are, while your reputation is merely what others think you are.

\- John Wooden, American coach

The best way to build character is to learn from your experiences or from the experiences of others by reading the books written by highly evolved people. The best place to buy books is on www.amazon.com.

RECOMMENDED READING

Dying To Be Me by Anita Moorjani
www.anitamoorjani.com

Proof of Heaven by Eben Alexander III M. D.
www.lifebeyonddeath.net

To Heaven and Back by Mary C. Neal
www.drmaryneal.com

My Journey to Heaven by Marvin J. Besteman and Lorilee Craker
www.myjourneytoheaven.com

Your Soul's Gift by Robert Schwartz
www.yoursoulsplan.com

Miracles Happen by Brian L. Weiss
www.brianweiss.com

The Only Way to Win by Jim Loehr
www.hpinstitute.com

The 15 Invaluable Laws of Growth by John C. Maxwell
www.johnmaxwell.com

CHARACTER DEVELOPMENT

The selected devices, known as "mind machines" are helpful for self-development by relaxing and reprogramming the mind. They are helpful for changing the character during meditation. Use kinesiology, also known as muscle testing, to determine which device will work best.

MIND MACHINE DEVICES
Radionic Orgone Box
Transparent Corp Beyond Being
NeuroSky MindSet
Zen Master Mind Machine

Appendix A: Best Websites

BEAUTY PRODUCT REVIEWS
www.truthinaging.com
www.makeupalley.com

HEALTH STORES
www.vitacost.com
www.iherb.com
www.longevitywarehouse.com
www.mynaturalmarket.com
www.toolsforwellness.com
www.jcrowsmarketplace.com

DIY BEAUTY INGREDIENTS
www.lotioncrafter.com
www.skinactives.com
www.makingcosmetics.com
www.bulkactives.com
www.organic-creations.com

CONCLUSION

I apologize for missing certain brands that offer top quality and healthy products. I tried the best that I could to list every single brand or product that I knew of that offers the best in quality and health. In the future, I hope to include even more brands that offer the best and most healthy products in the world. Please contact me if you know of such brands and products, as I will review them, and list them in future editions of this book.

If you are a company that offers high-quality, natural, and healthy products then please contact me on my website www.dianapolska.com and write a short description of the product you would like to present for review. Please include exact ingredient contents or construction, and a description of the benefits of the product and why it is better than any other products in its category; why is it the "best of the best"? Please also provide me with a publishable paragraph that I can use if your product gets selected to be included in future editions of *Perfect 10 Product Picks*. To reiterate, please include the following when contacting me with a product for review:
- Ingredients/construction
- Benefits of the product
- Why is it the "best of the best"?
- Publishable paragraph

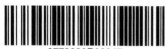

Made in the USA
San Bernardino, CA
15 December 2013